Breathe & Bloom 4

Flower Patterns

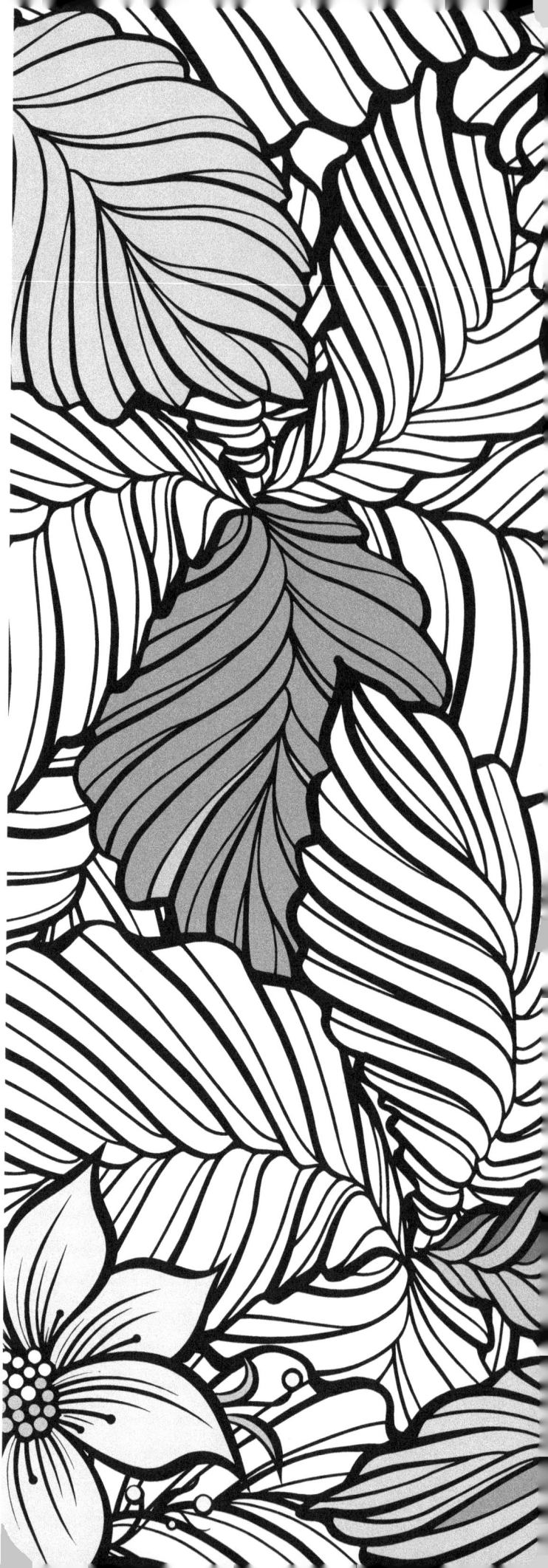

Breathe & Bloom 4

Flower Patterns

A Global Floral Coloring Journey

for Calm & Peace.

Rosa Englerton

How to Use
this Book

Hi and thank you for joining us in this journey of peace and relaxation.

This coloring book combines natural imagery with breathing exercises that help you return to return to ease and relaxation.

Help yourself affirms the right to rest and reset. Shifts your focus from being fixed to feeling free and elevated. Support yourself with mental clarity during chaotic moments. Reaffirm your will with agency during stress. Take a safe internal refuge. Restore your inner strength and balance.

The book has ten sections followed by ten-large size paintable flowers.

Start by reading the breathing exercise. Meditate on it for a few minutes, and start your breathing. Close your eyes. Look for the light of the Creator. Relax and put yourself in His hands.

Now you are ready to take your favourite coloring pencils, crayons, or markers, and let yourself flow into the flower and the colors. Be free. Imagine you are in the garden of Paradise. You are in control. The flower is your friend and is allowing you to give it the colors you want. Paint the background with patterns, or draw your own flowers.

When you are done painting, look at the flower, and do the breathing exercise again. If you have time, take a walk in the park. Look at the greenery, look at the flowers, see the colors in the world that surround you.

Breathe.

Everything is ok.
You are stronger now.

God Bless you!

Scent Imagination

Look at the flower on the opposite page.

- Close your eyes
- Imagine the scent of this flower
- Imagine its color

The 5-4-3-2-1 Grounding Moment

What to do:
Pause and name:

- 5 things you can see

....

....

....

....

....

- 4 things you can touch

....

....

....

- 3 things you can hear

....

....

- 2 things you can smell

....

....

- 1 thing you can are grateful for

....

Affirmation **Quote**

With each breath, I soften into peace.

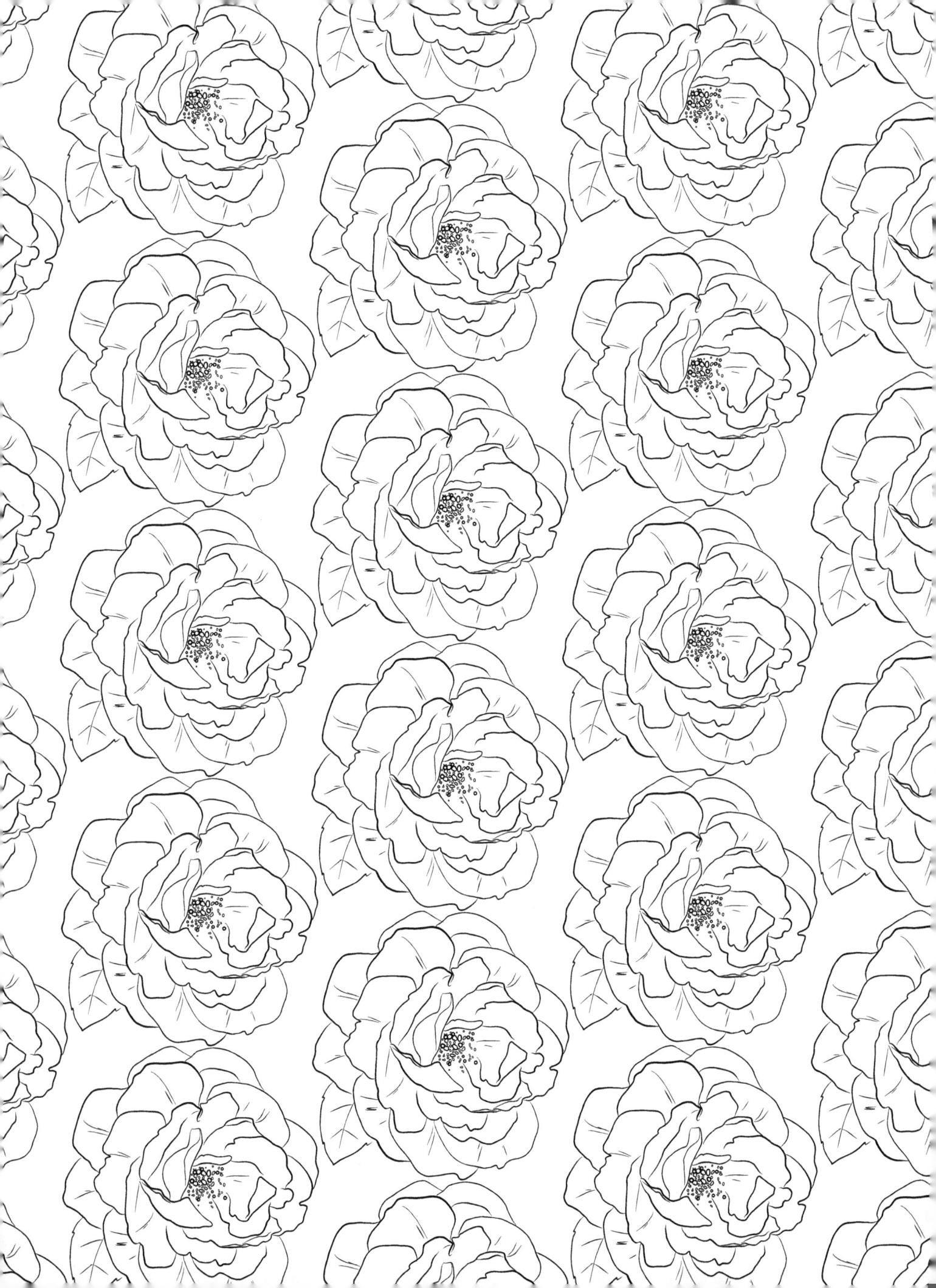

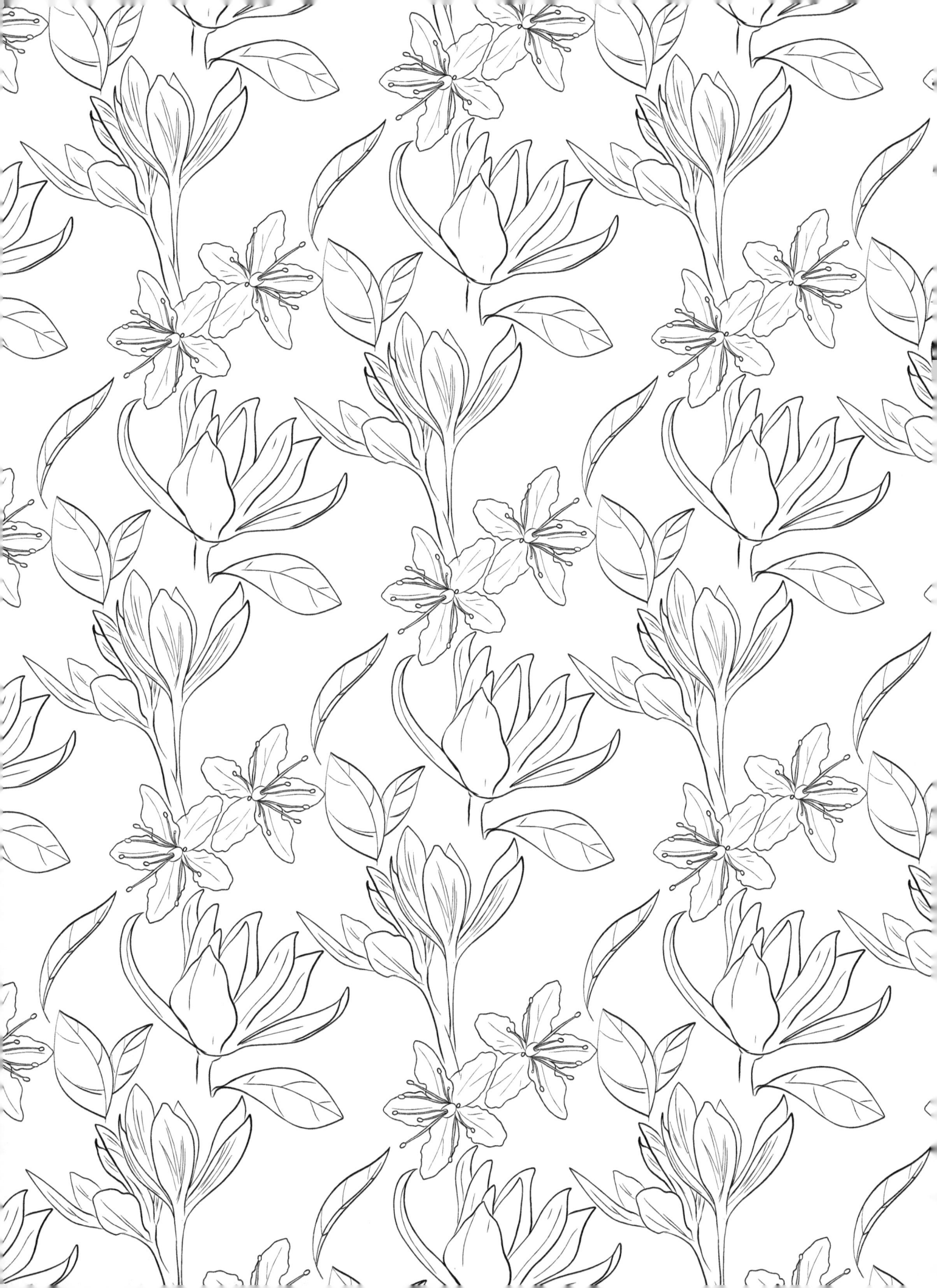

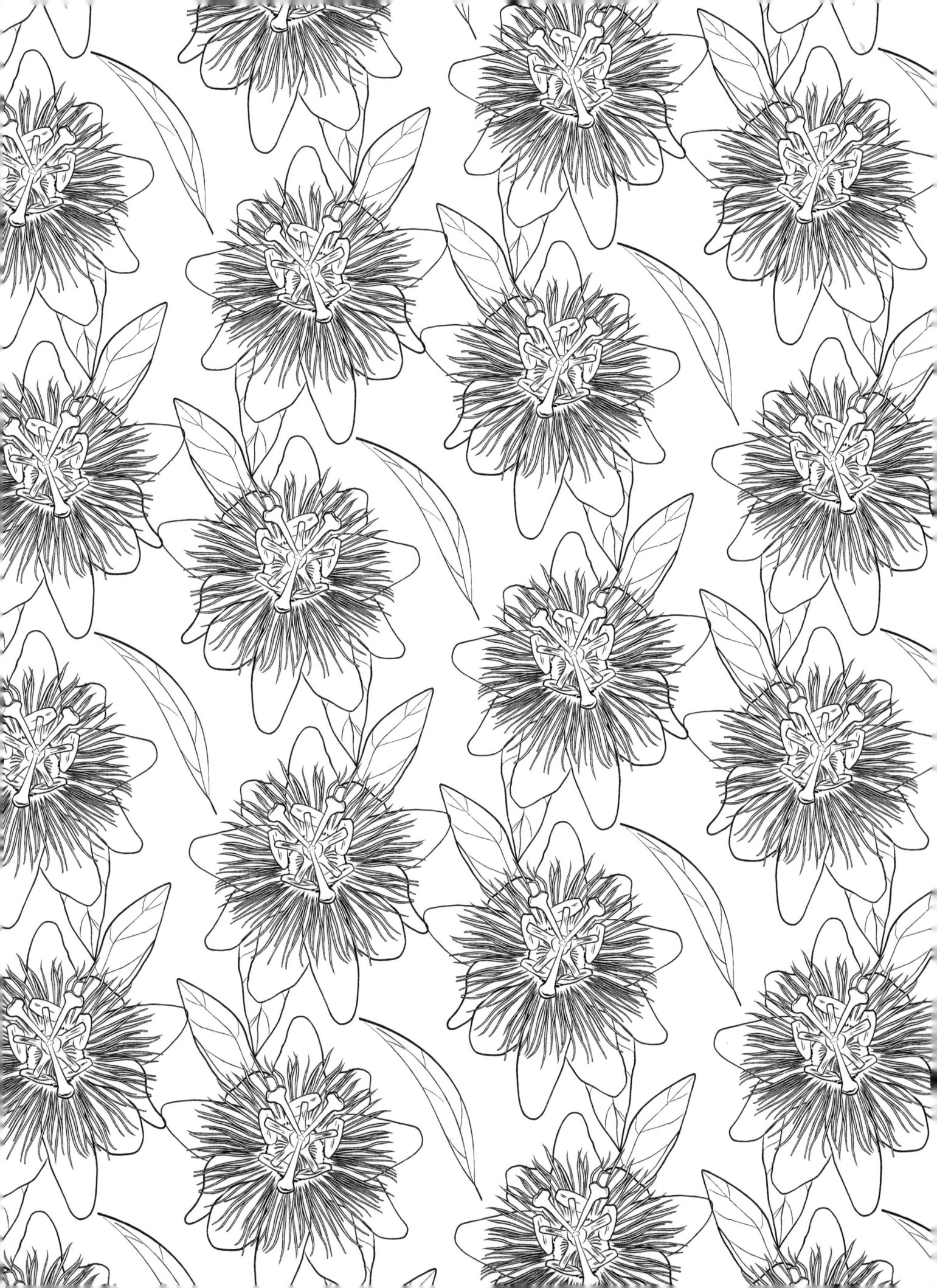

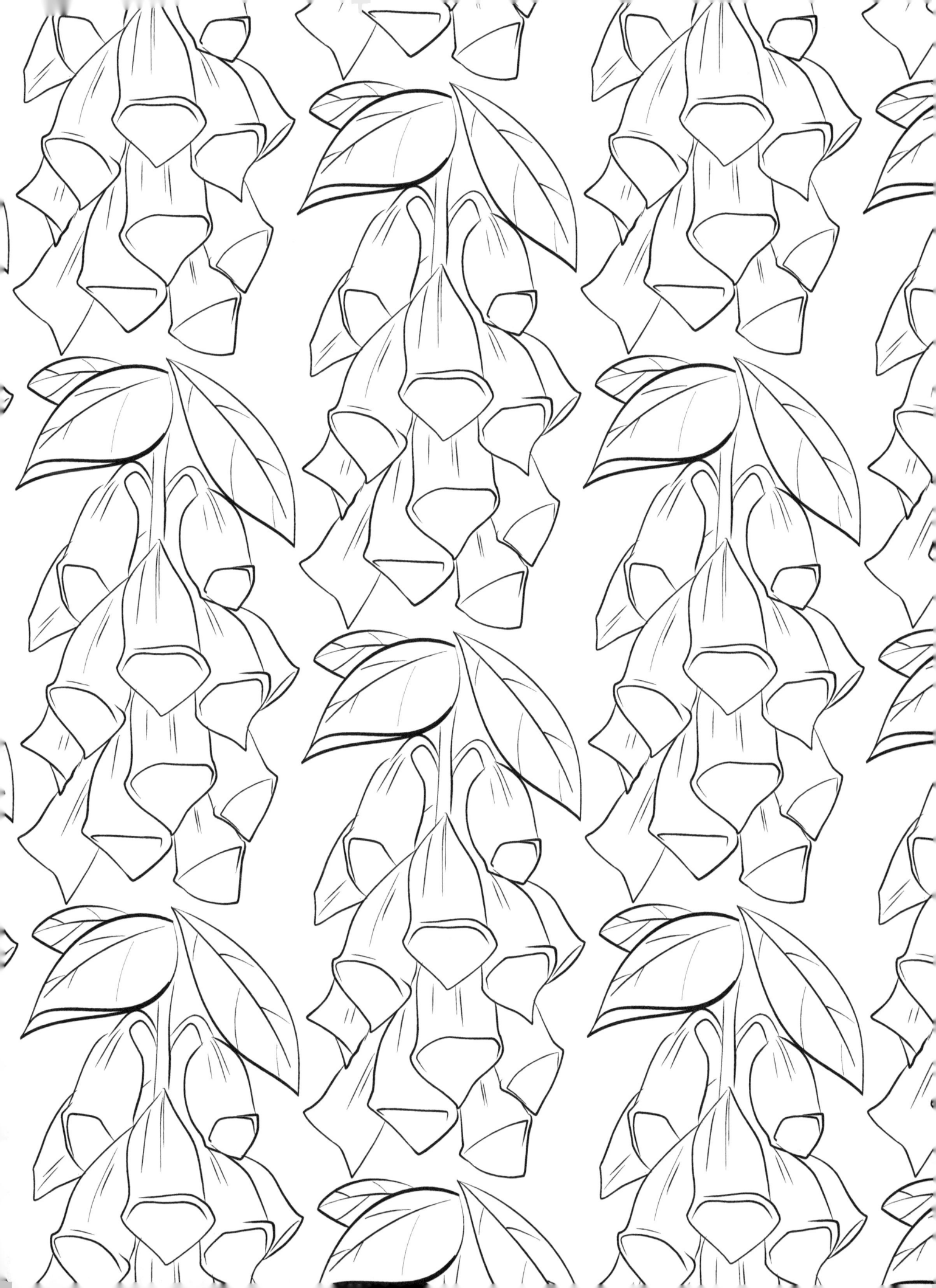

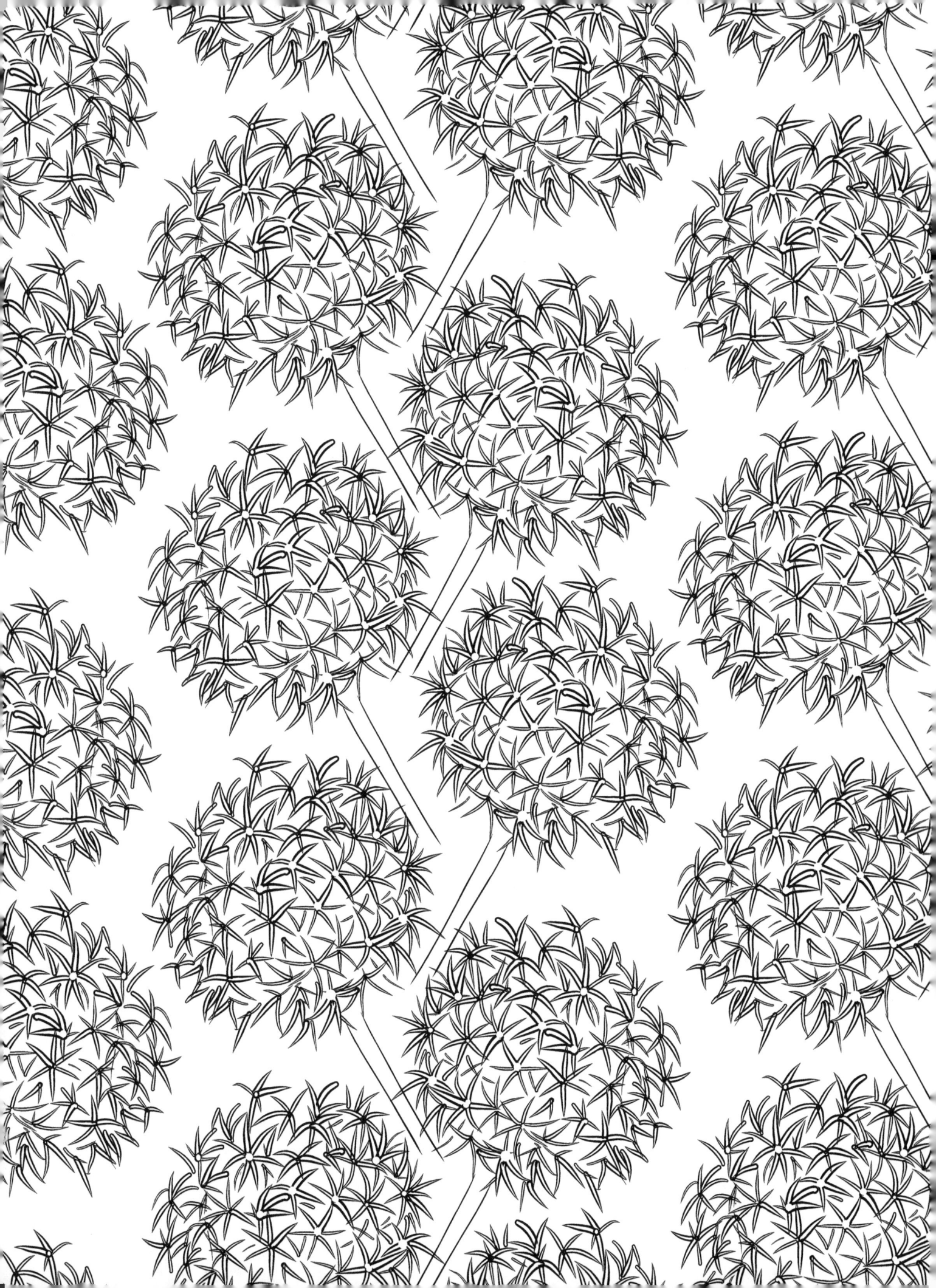

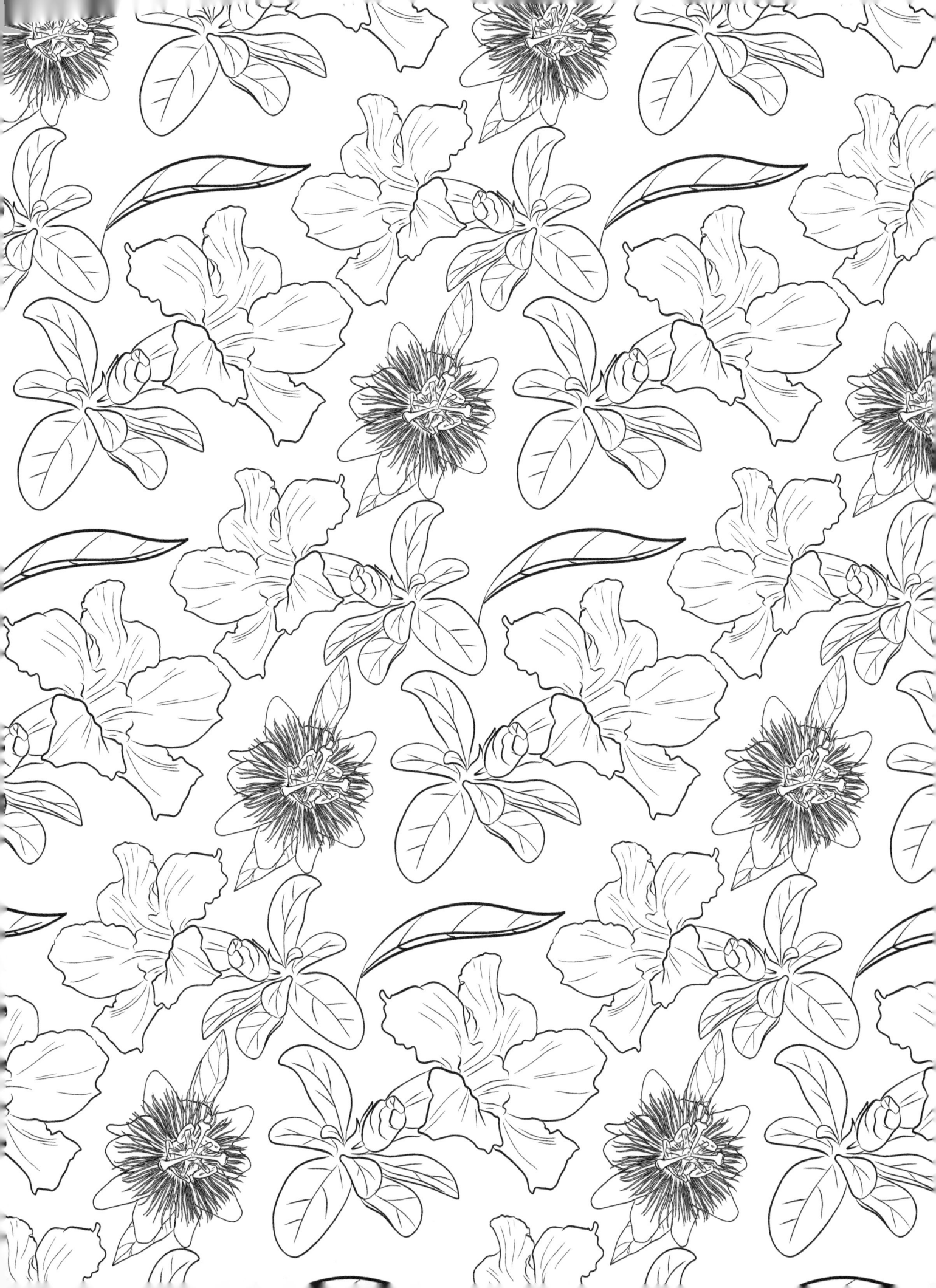

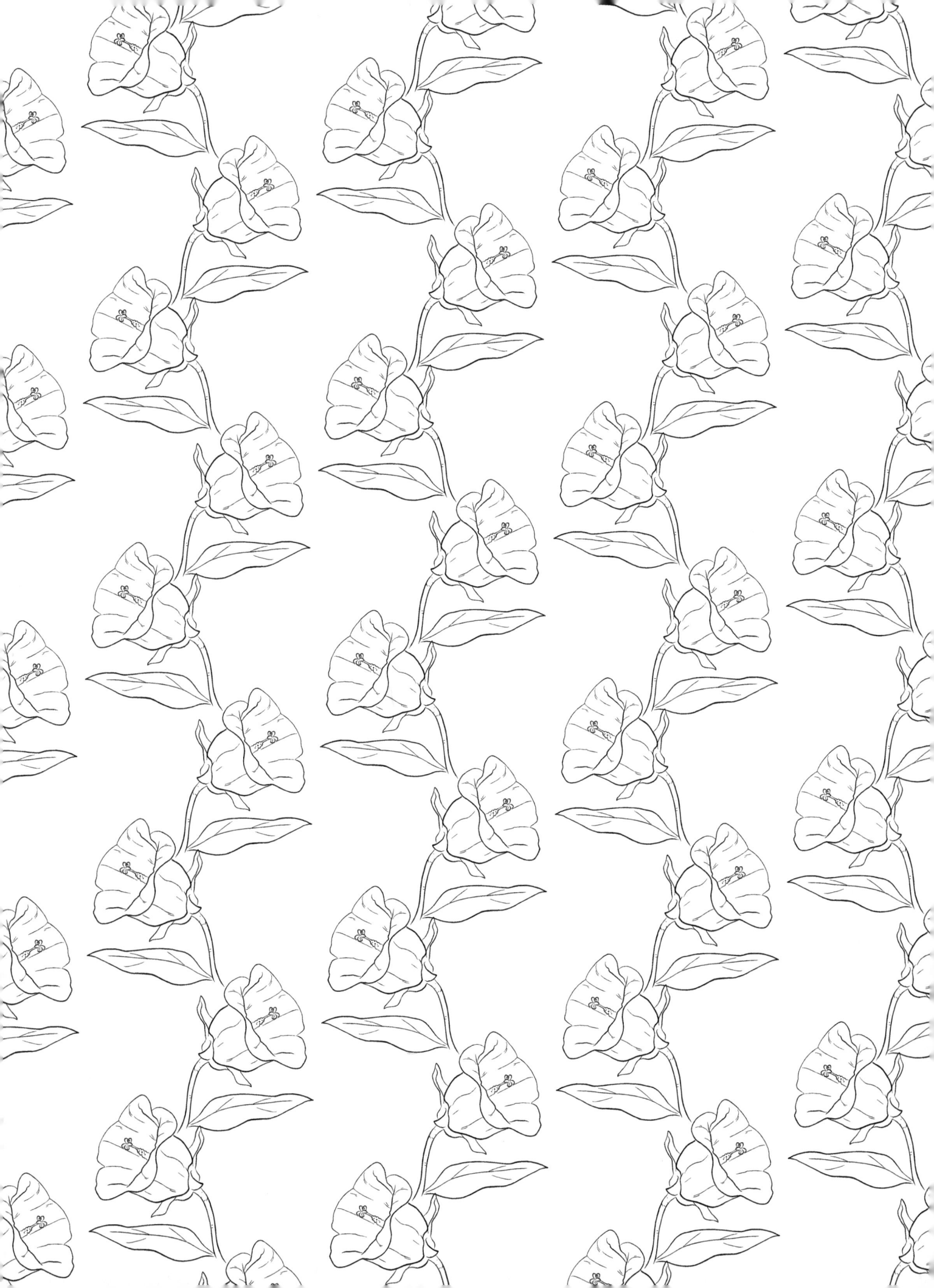

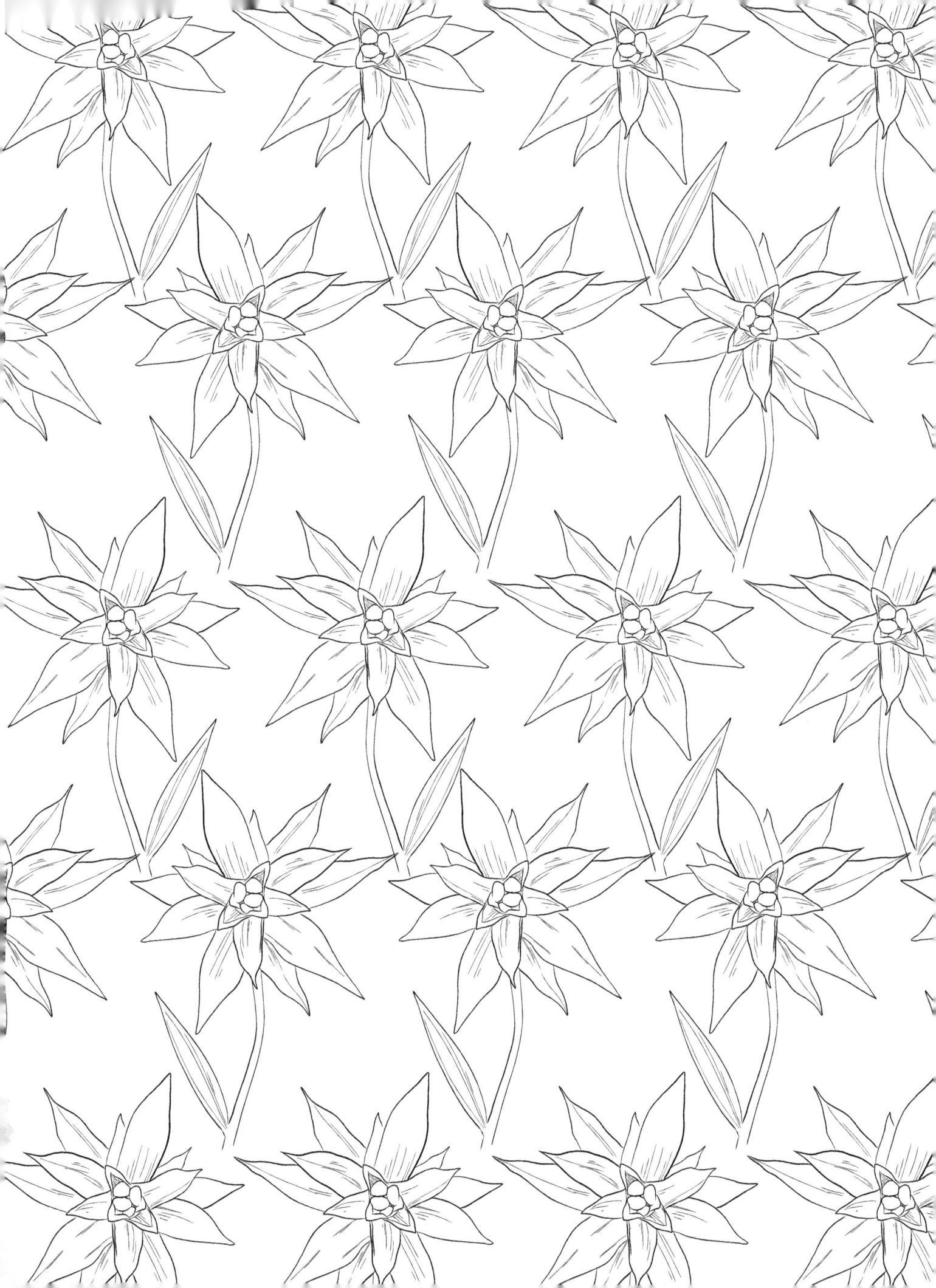

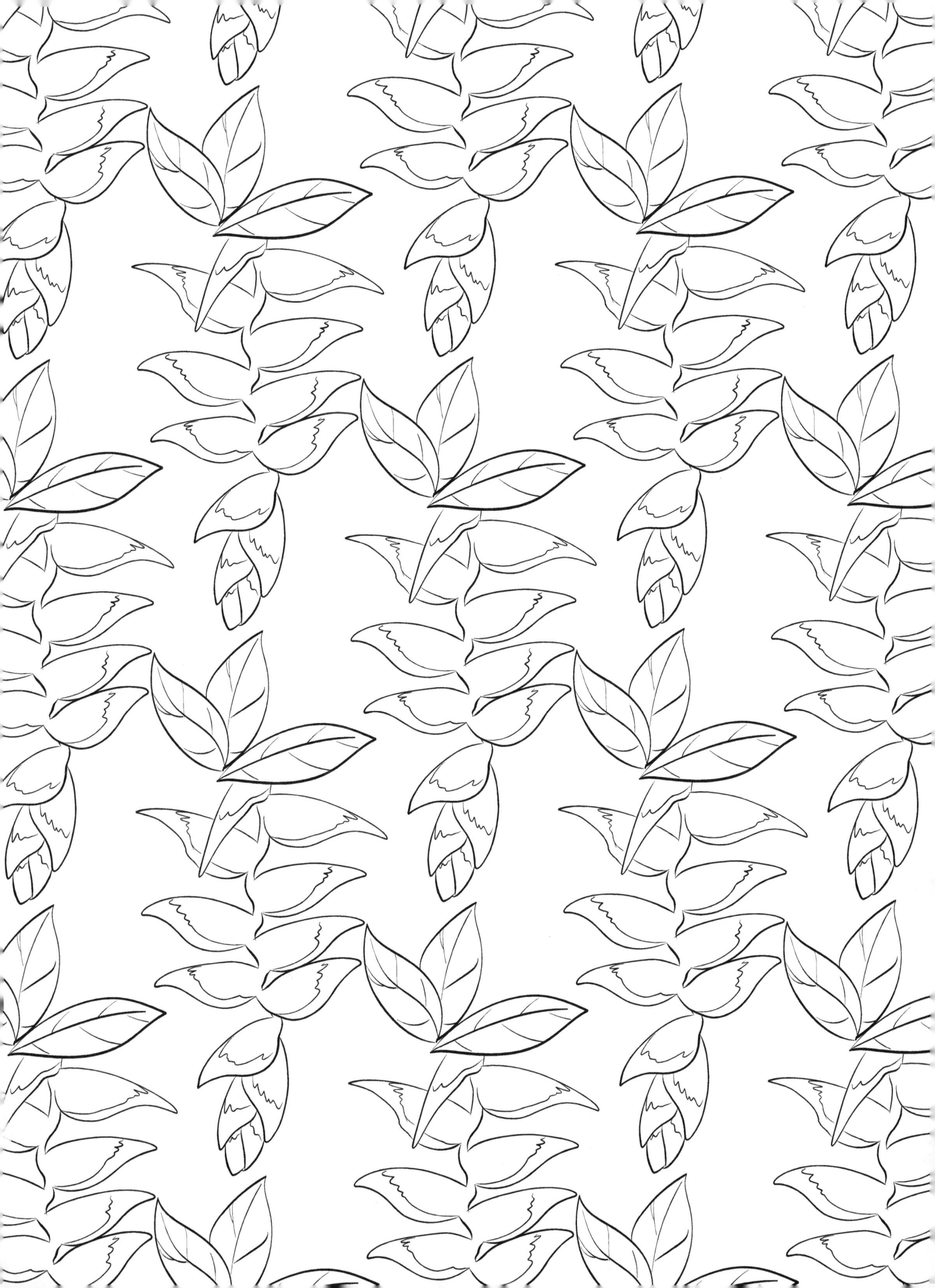

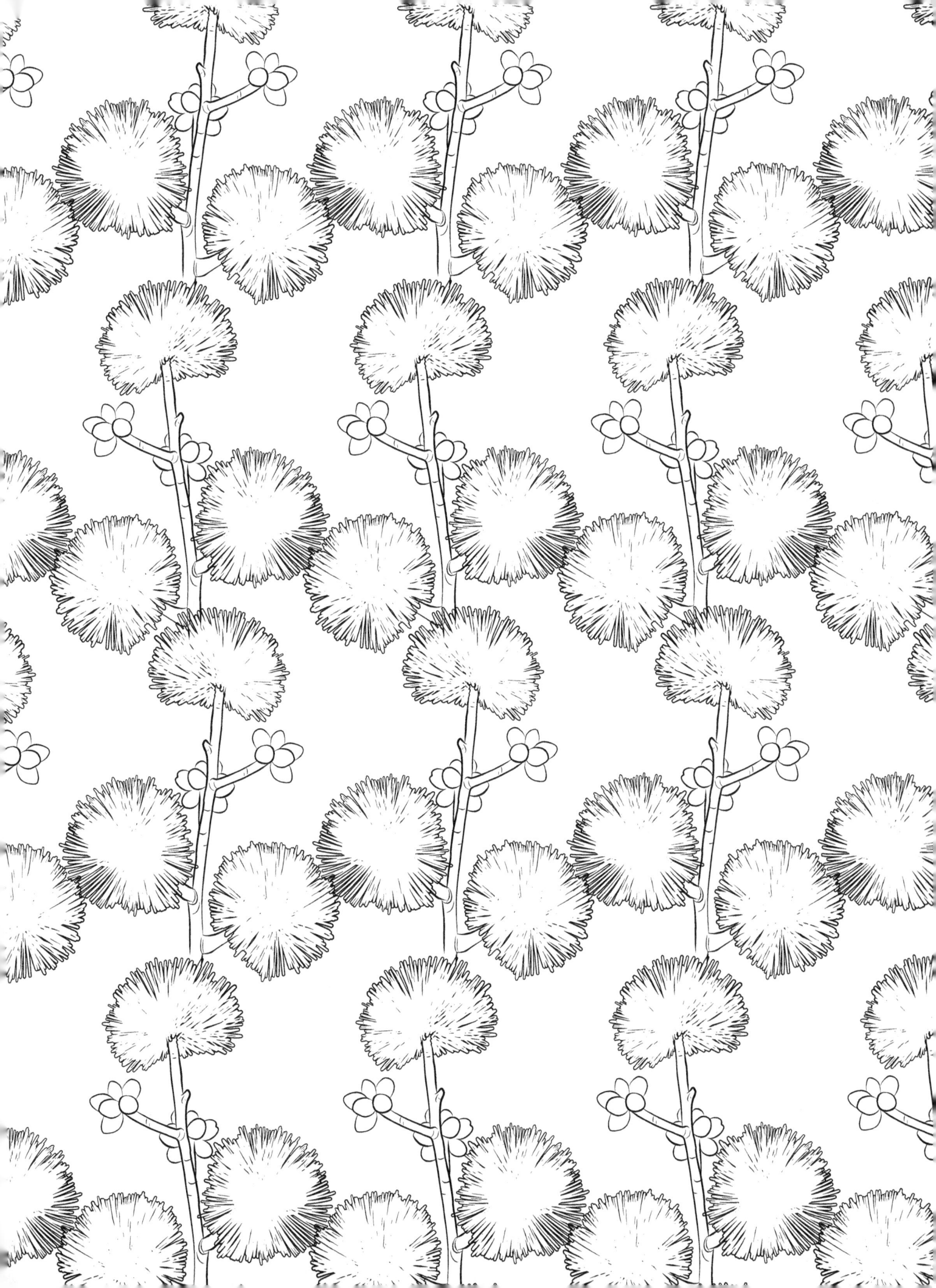

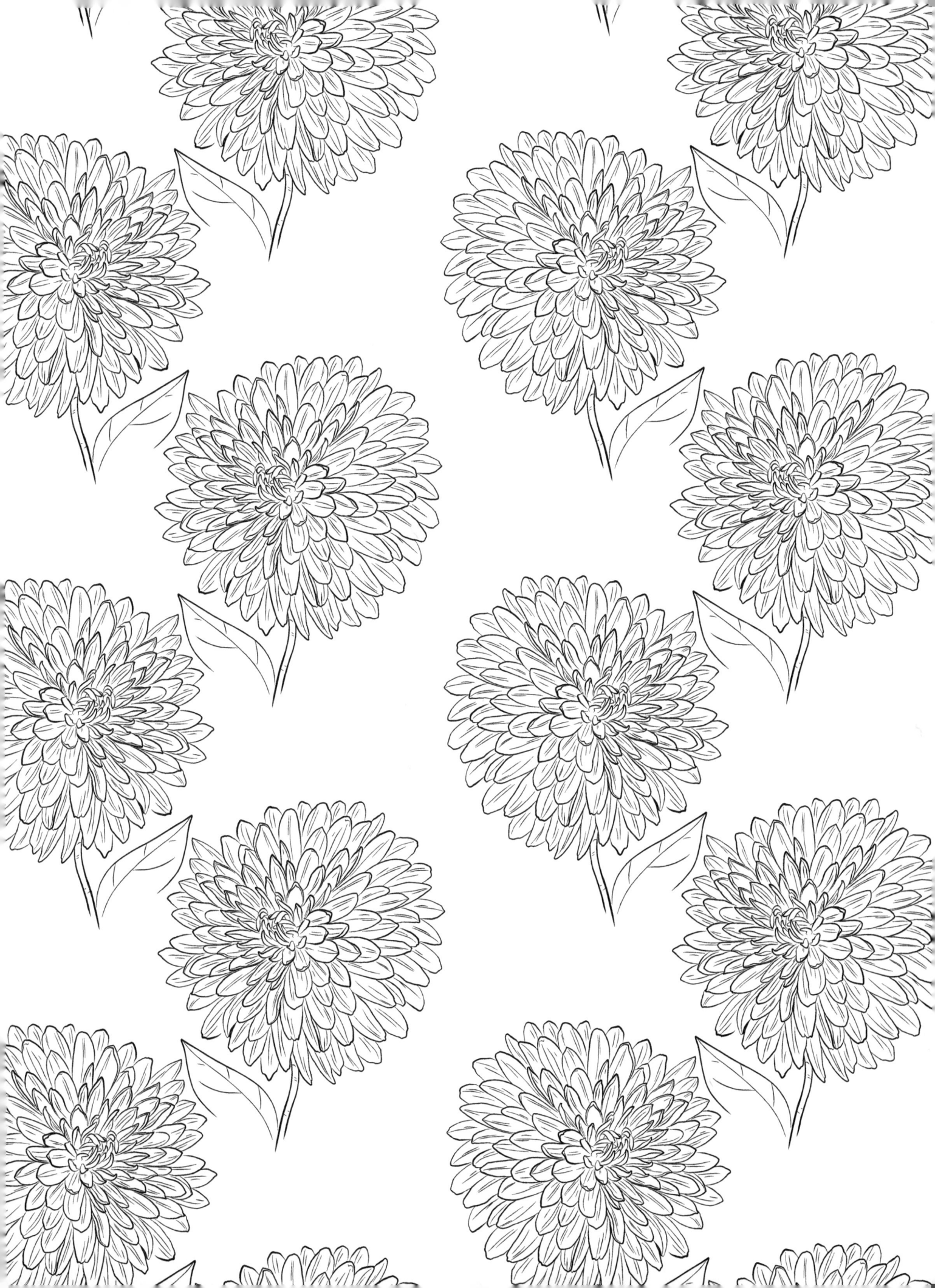

Scent Imagination

Look at the flower on the opposite page.

- Close your eyes
- Imagine the scent of this flower
- Imagine its color

Petal Drop Visualization

Close your eyes and imagine a single petal floating
slowly down with each exhale. Let each falling petal carry away
a stressful thought.

Affirmation
Quote

I am anchored in this moment. Nothing else matters right now.

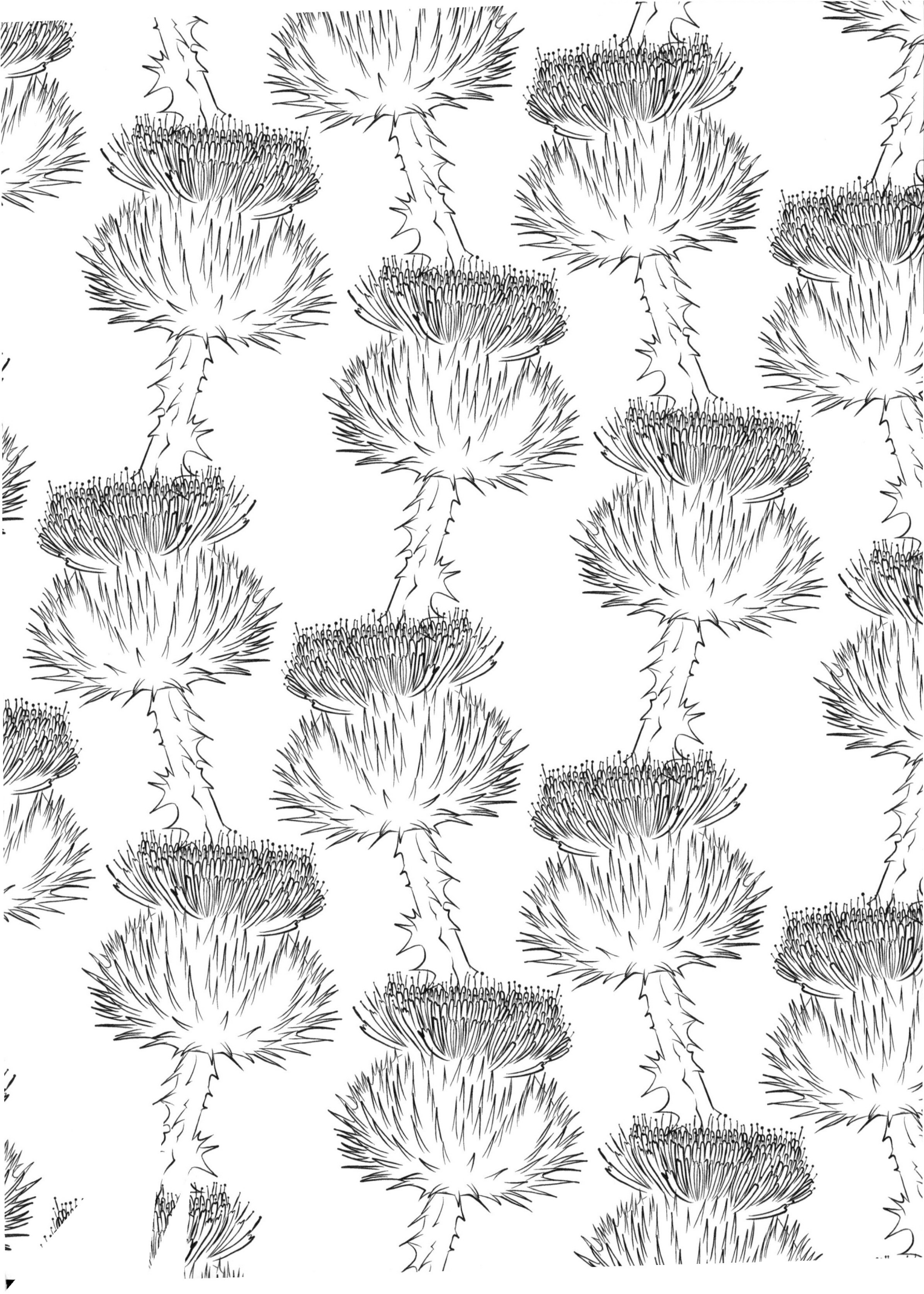

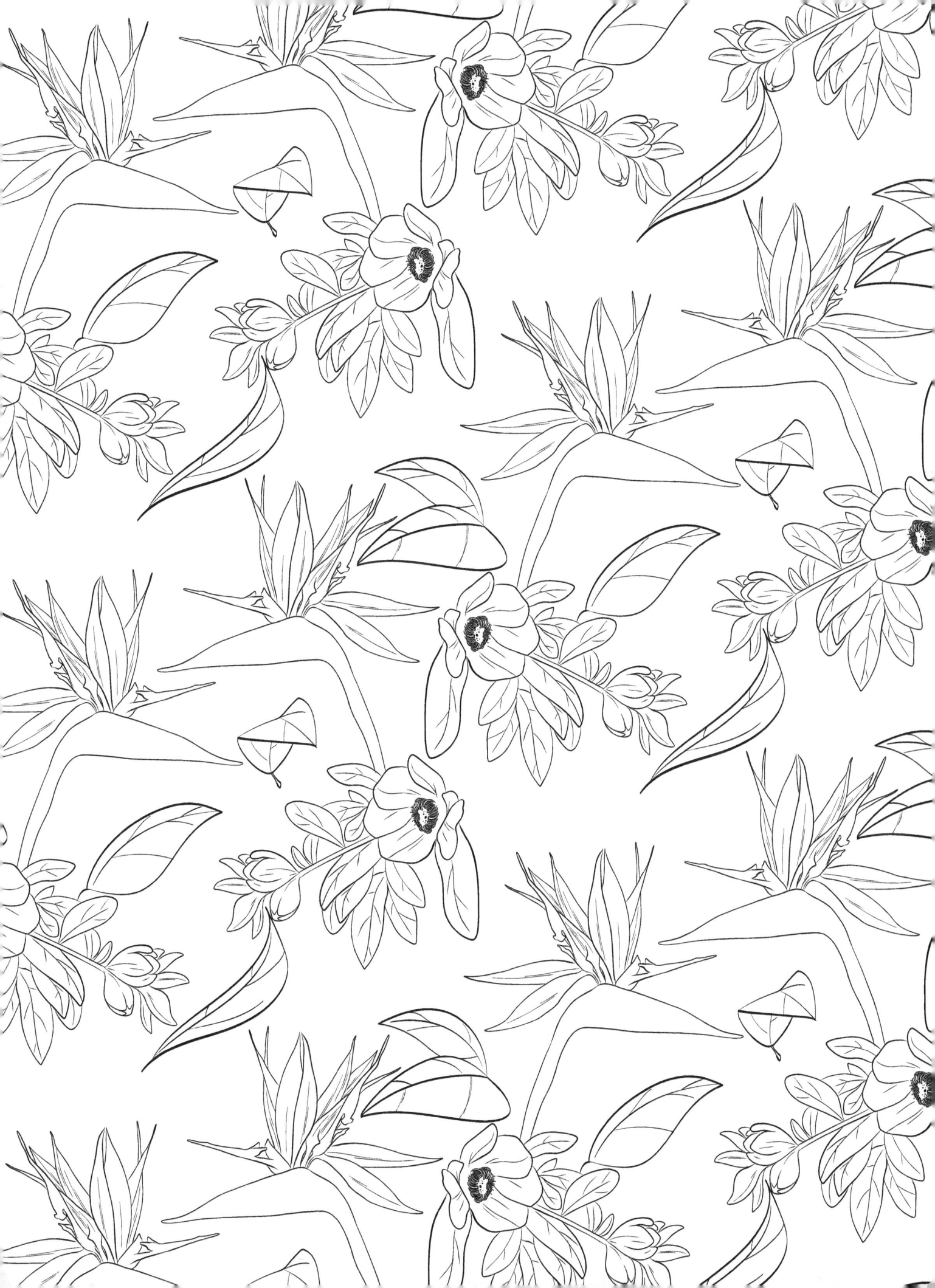

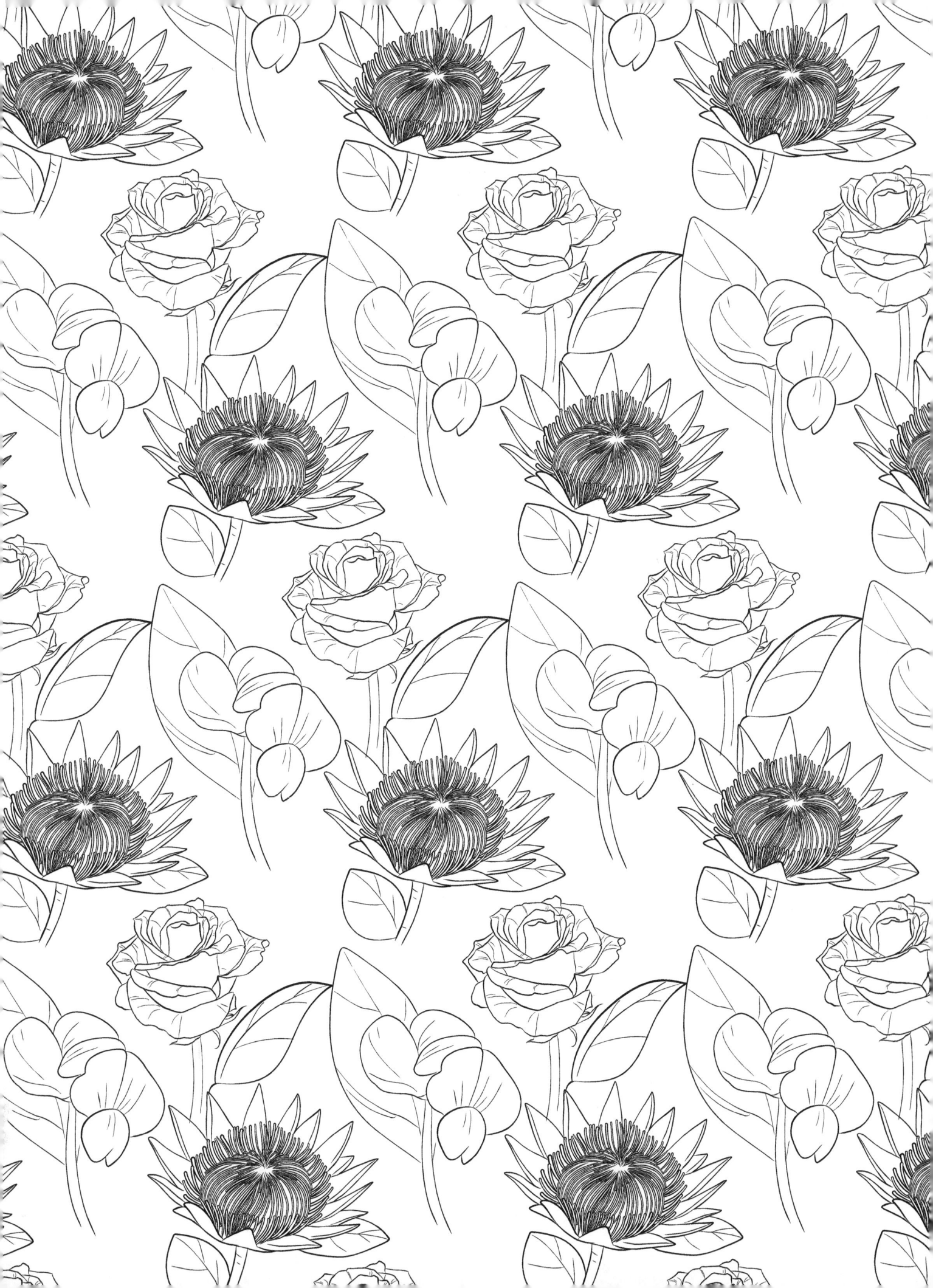

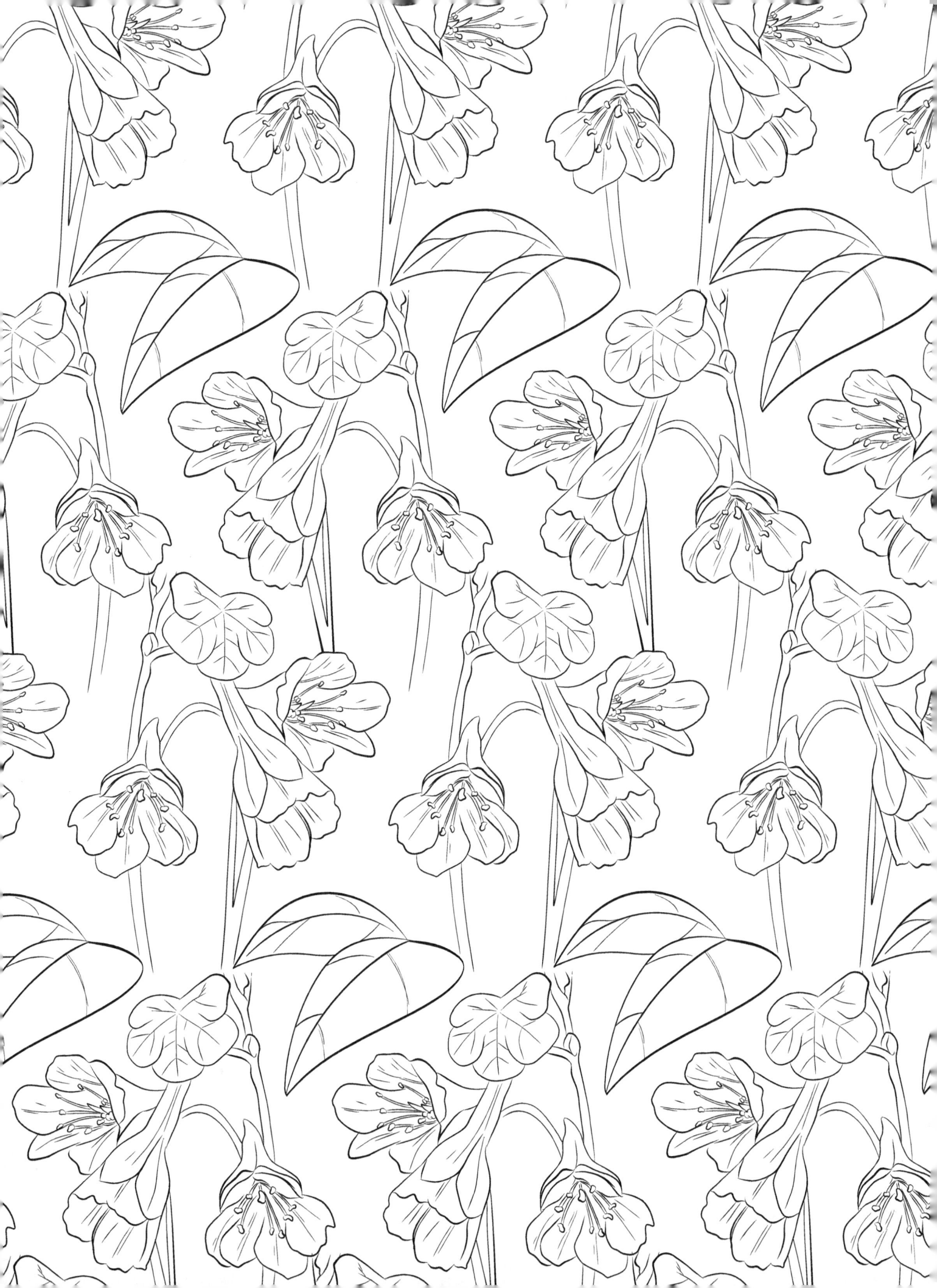

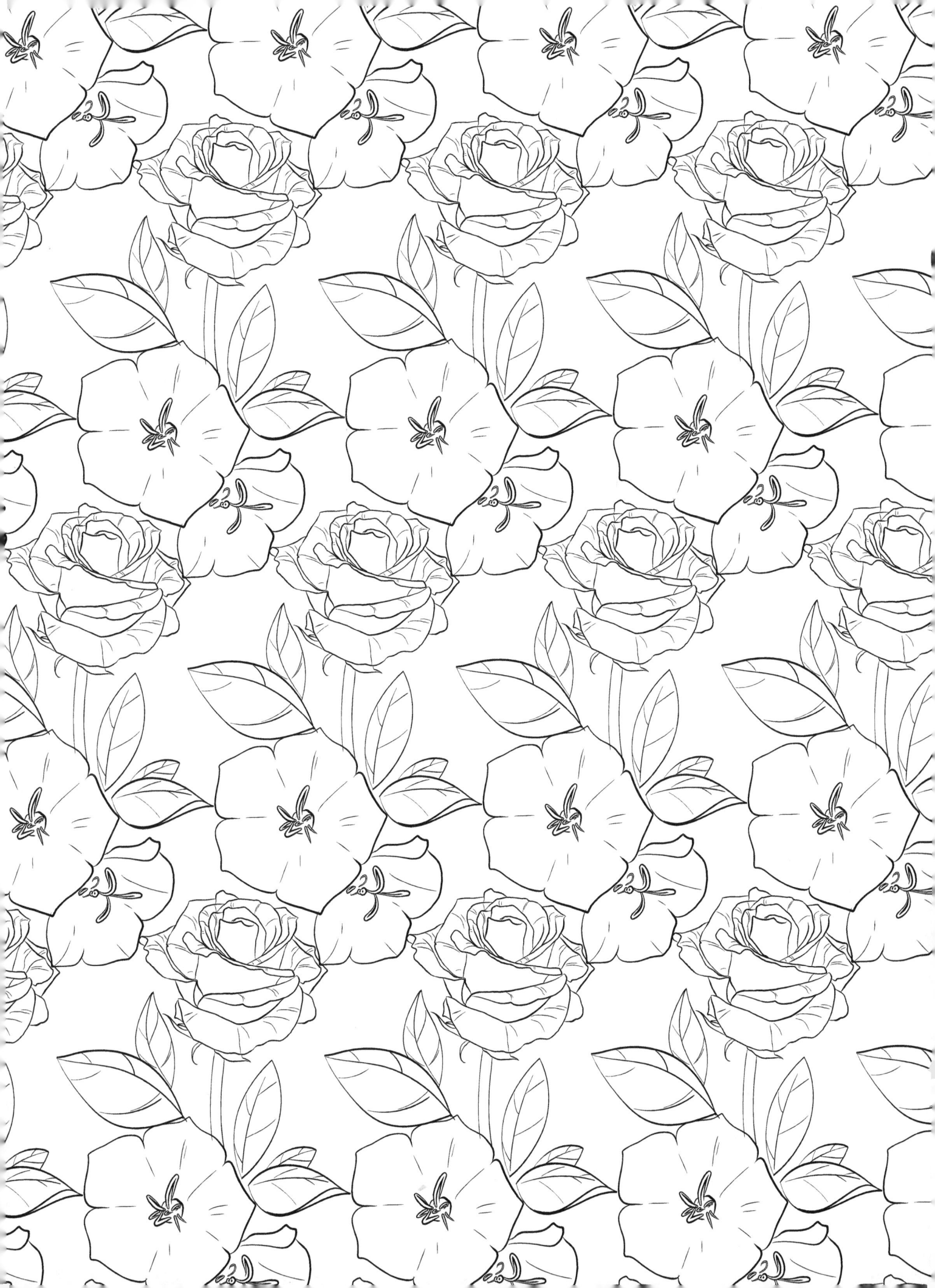

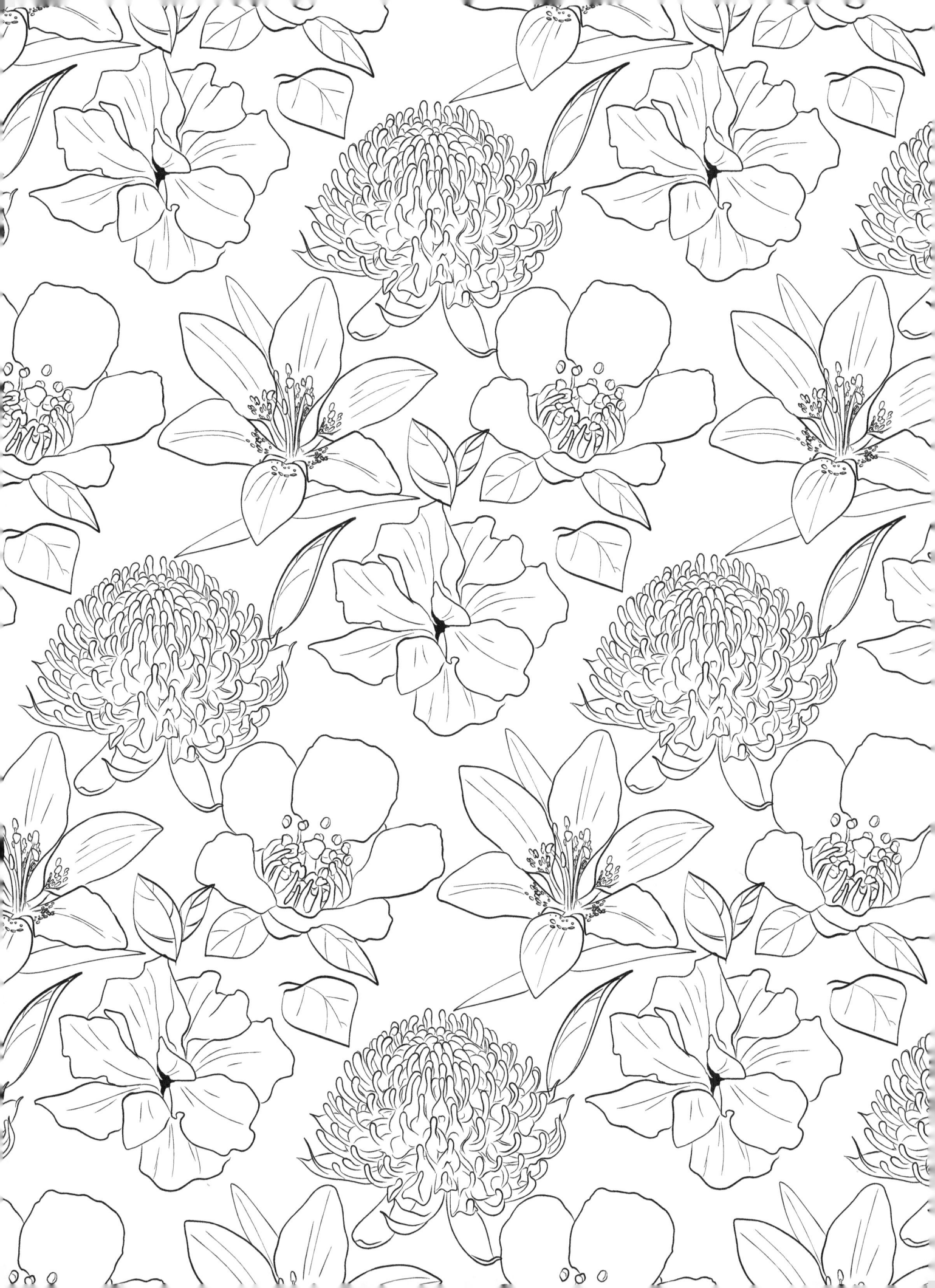

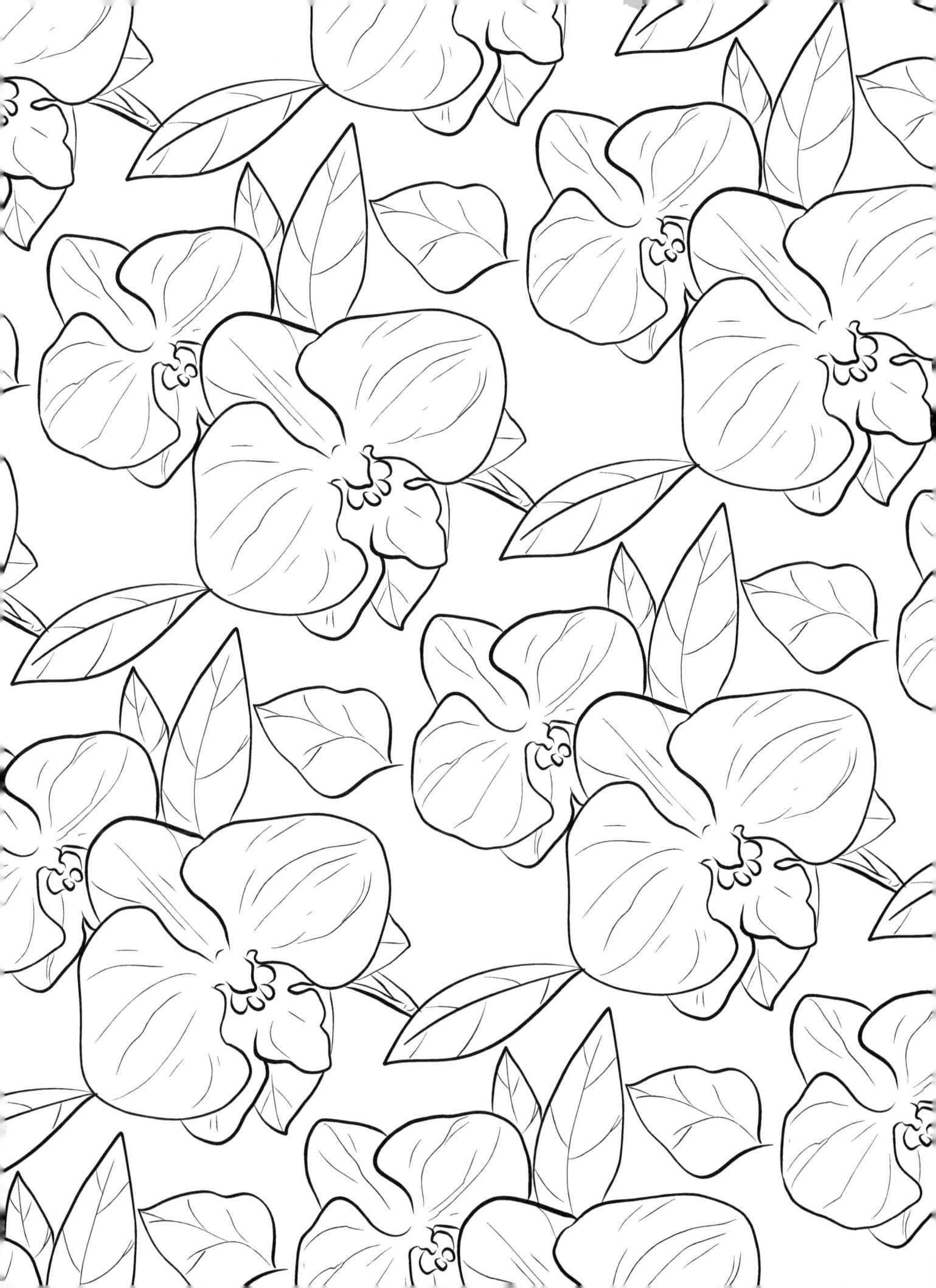

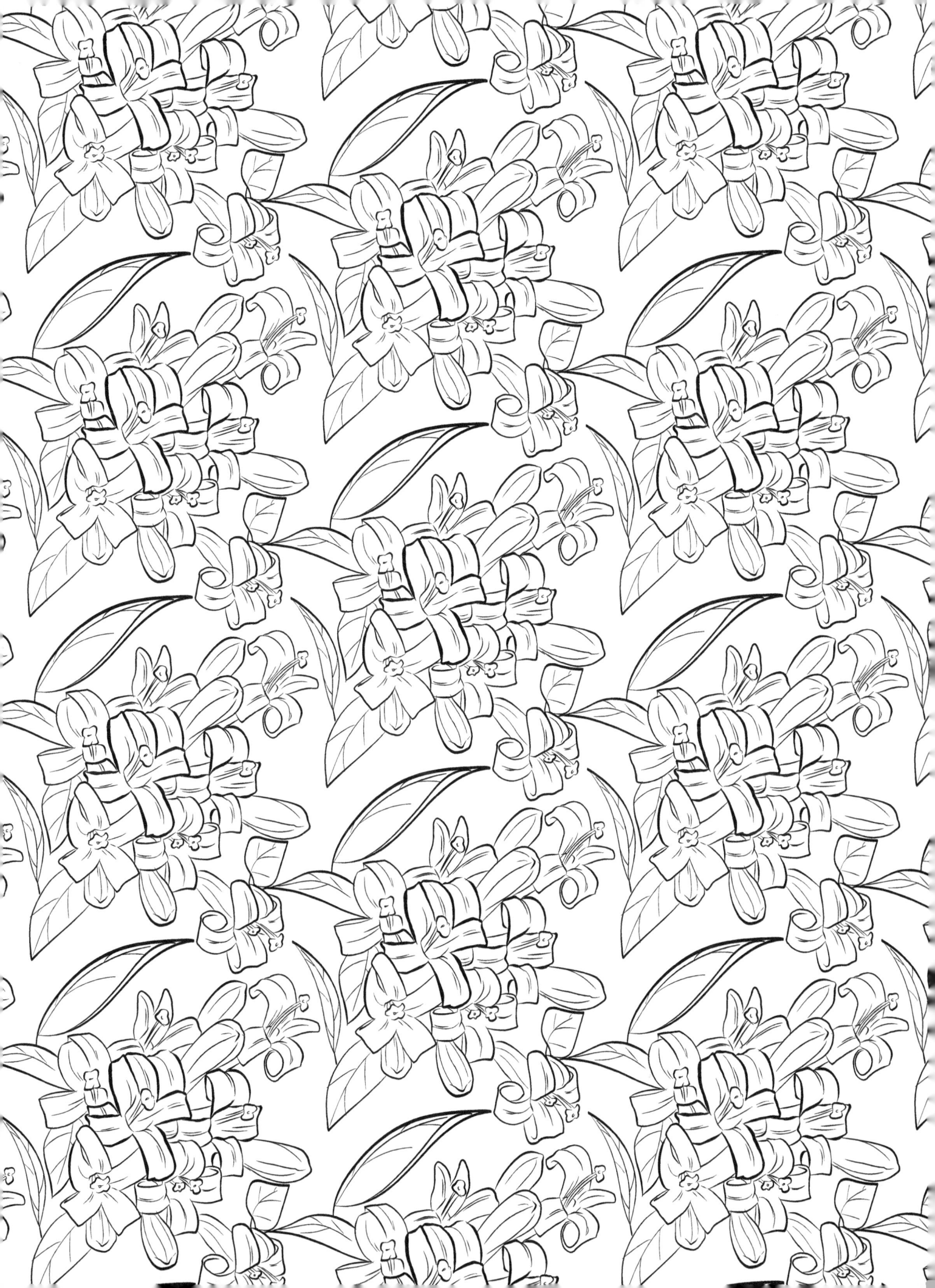

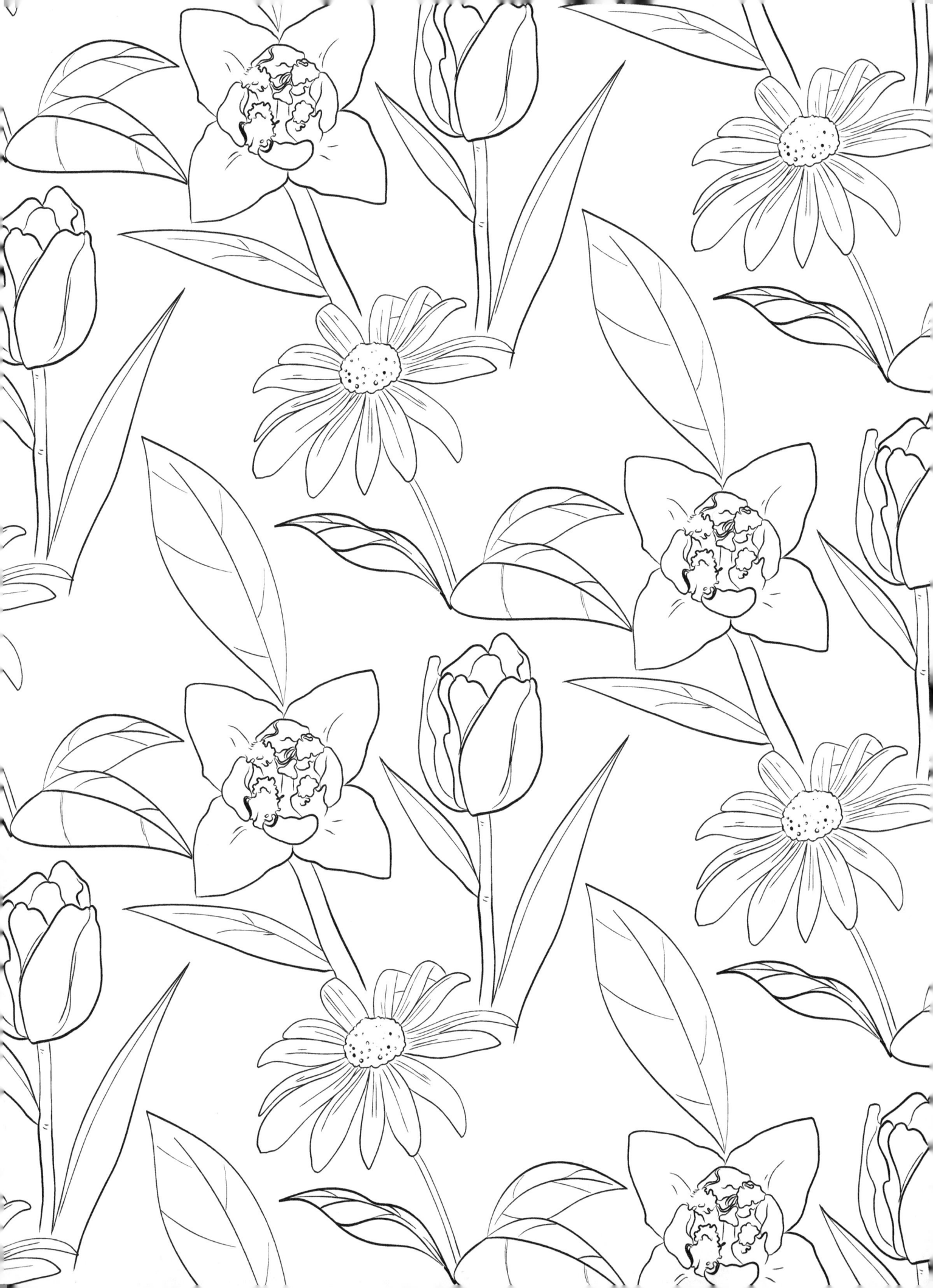

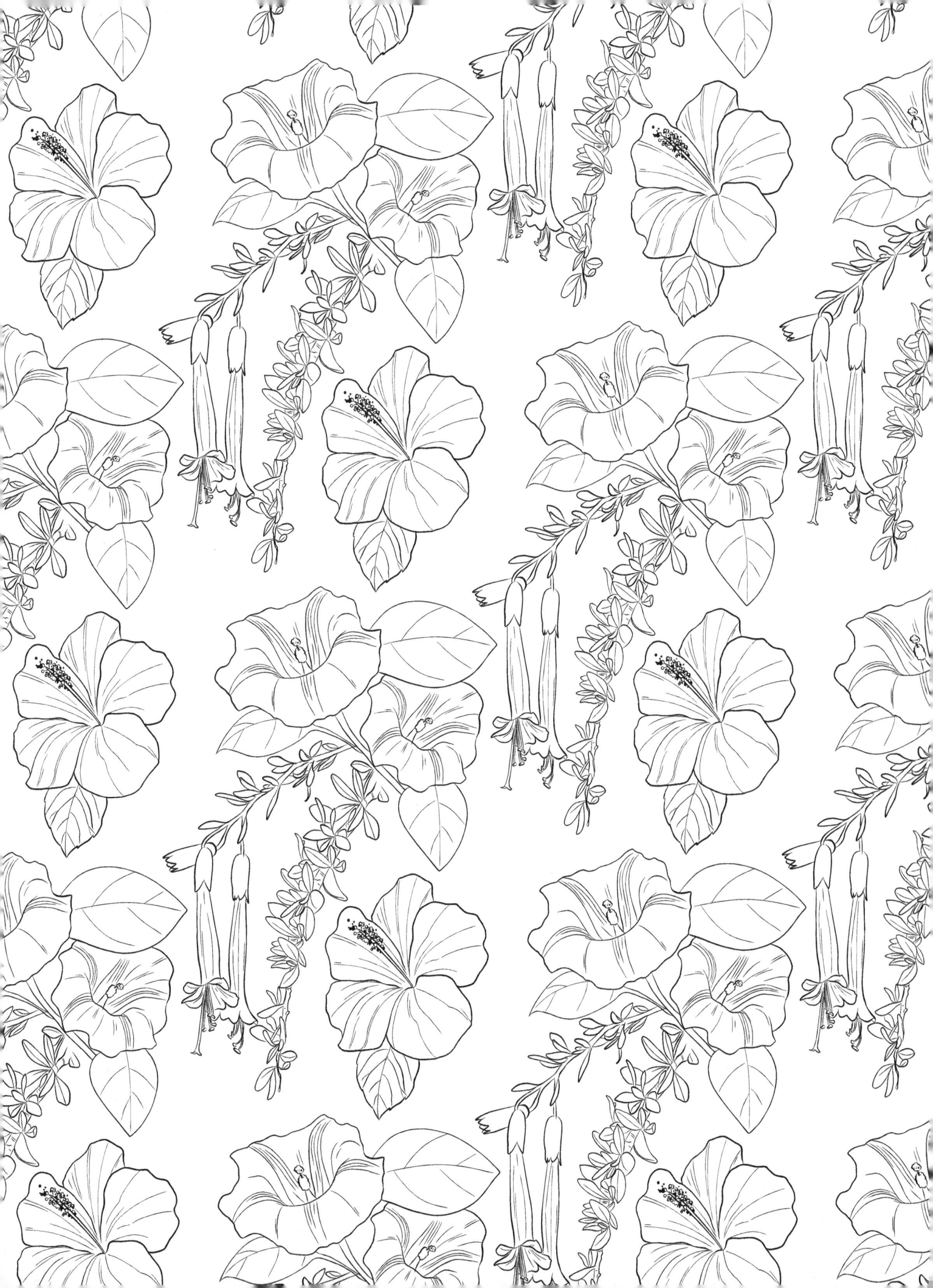

Scent Imagination

Look at the flower on the opposite page.

- Close your eyes
- Imagine the scent of this flower
- Imagine its color

Hand on Heart, Breath in Peace

- Place your hand on your chest. Inhale deeply and say in your mind:
  "I am safe."
- Exhale and think: *"I am calm."*
- Repeat 3–5 times.

Affirmation Quote

As I exhale, I let go of what I cannot control.

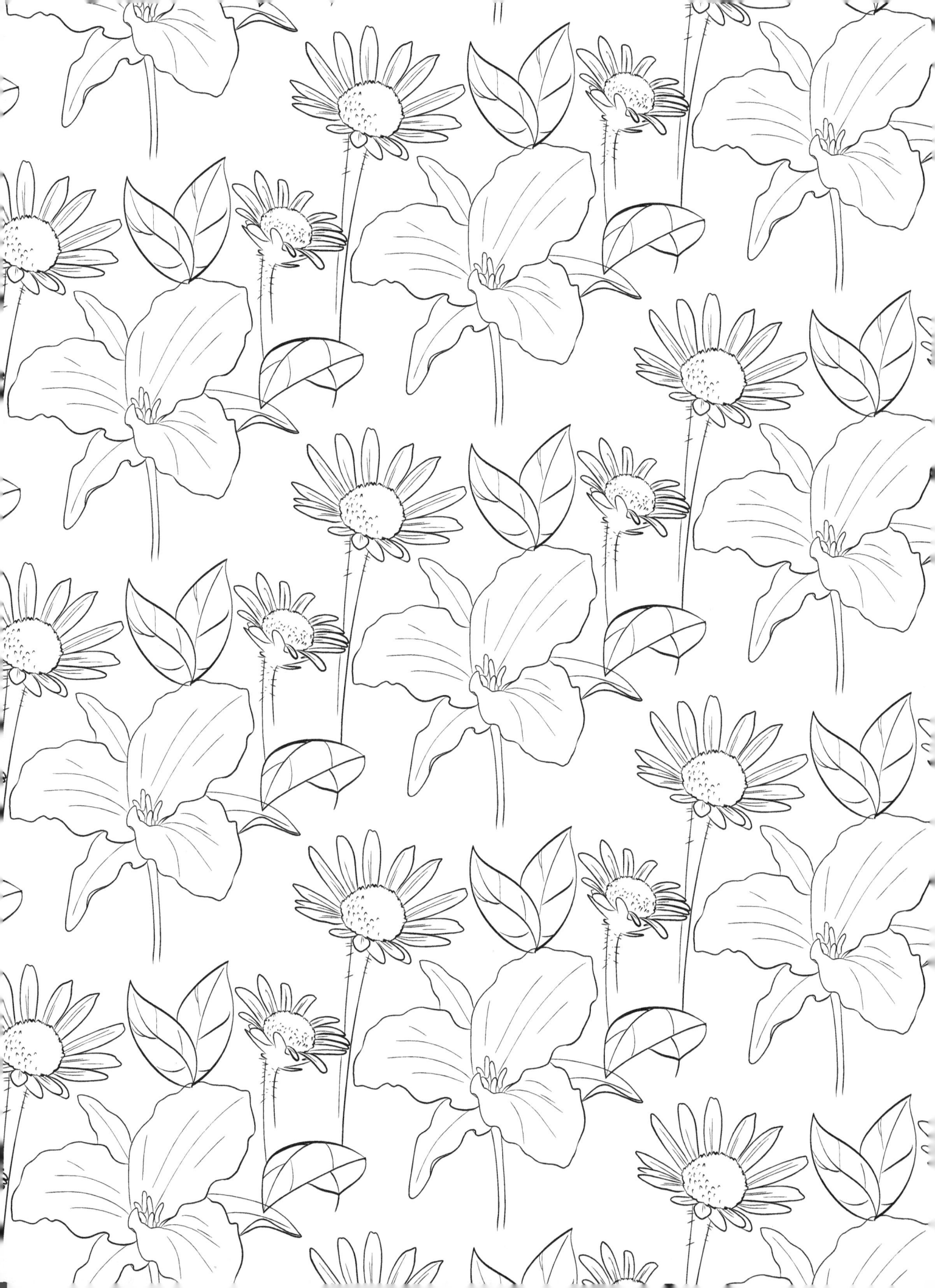

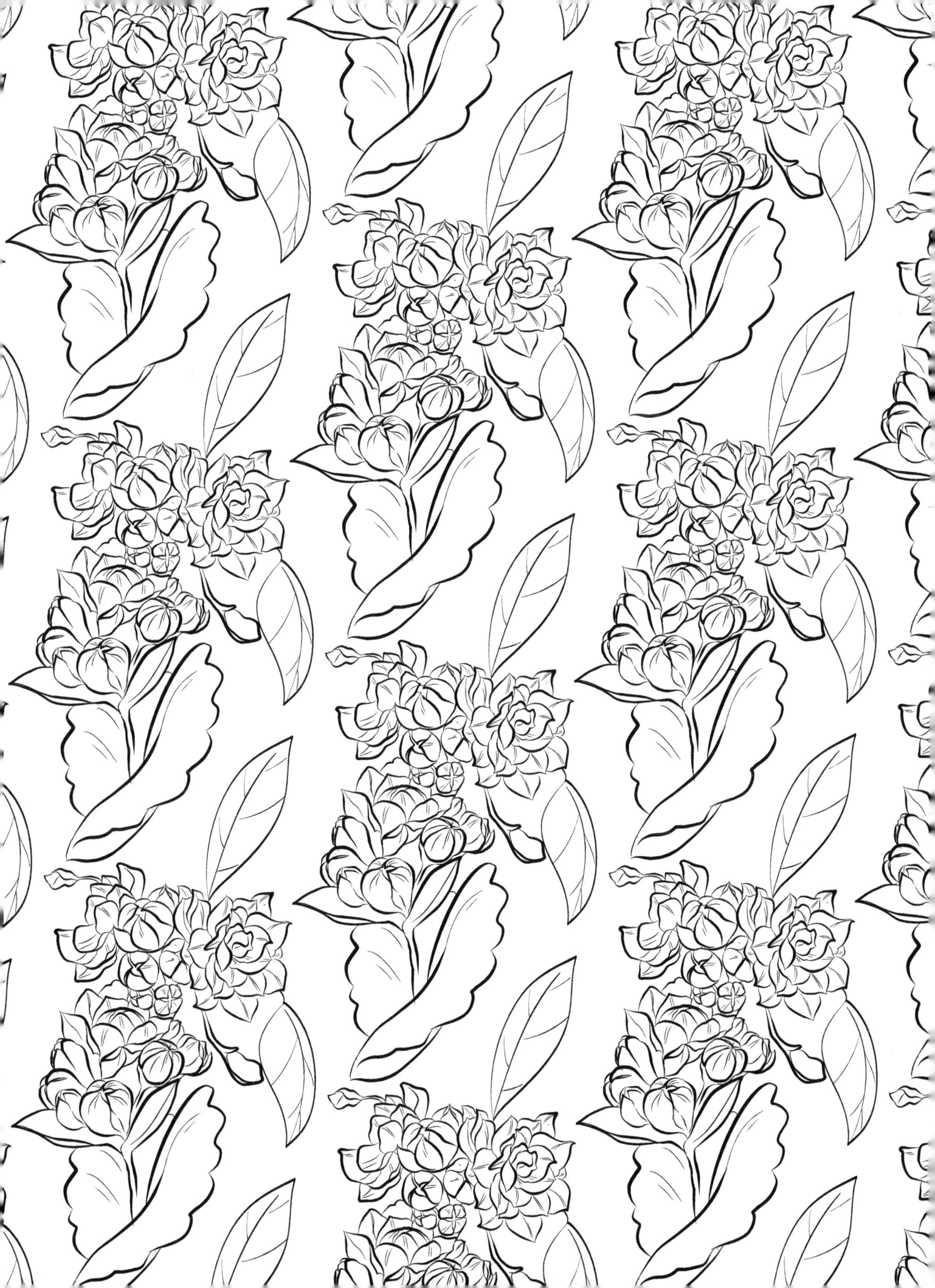

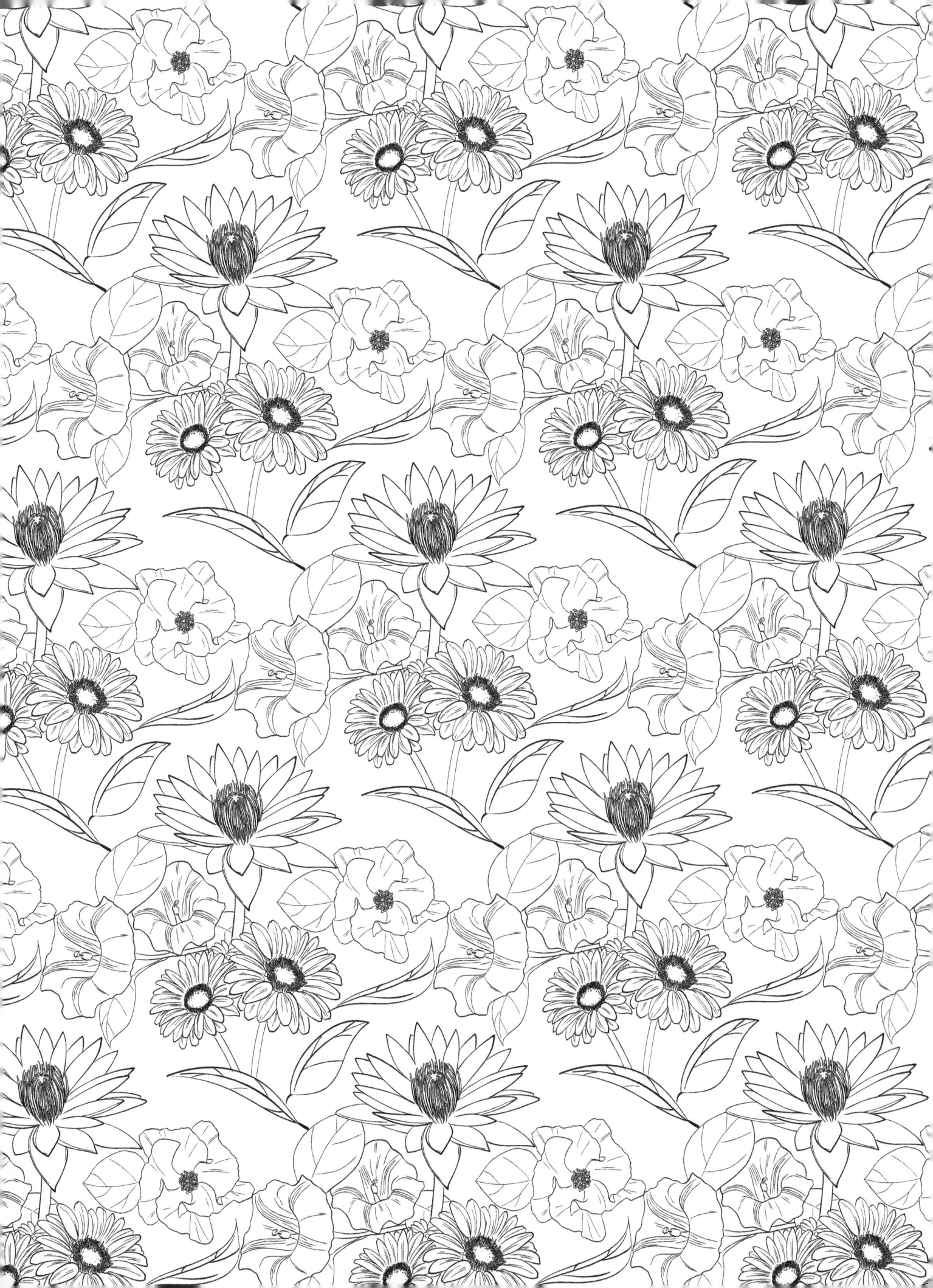

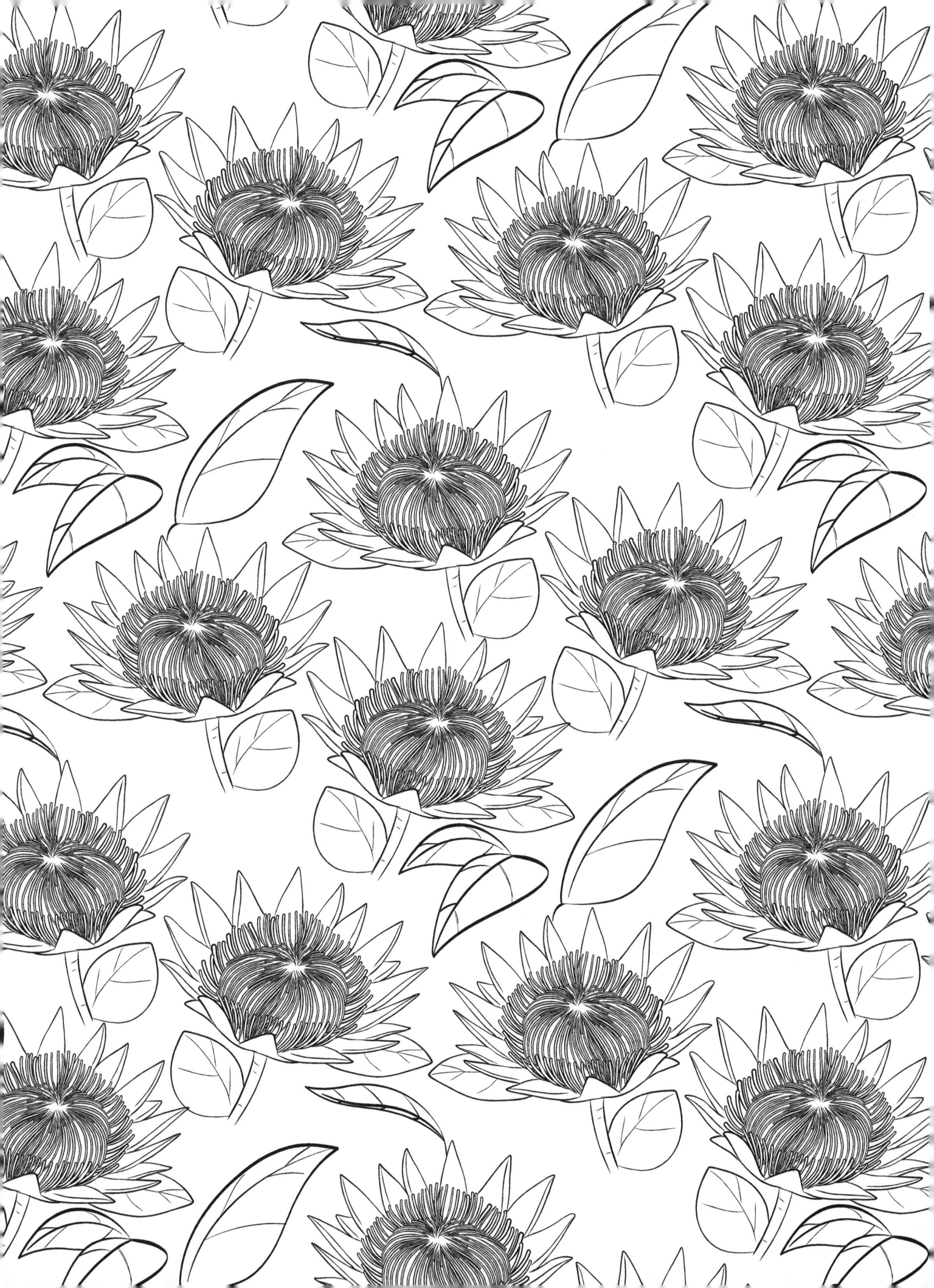

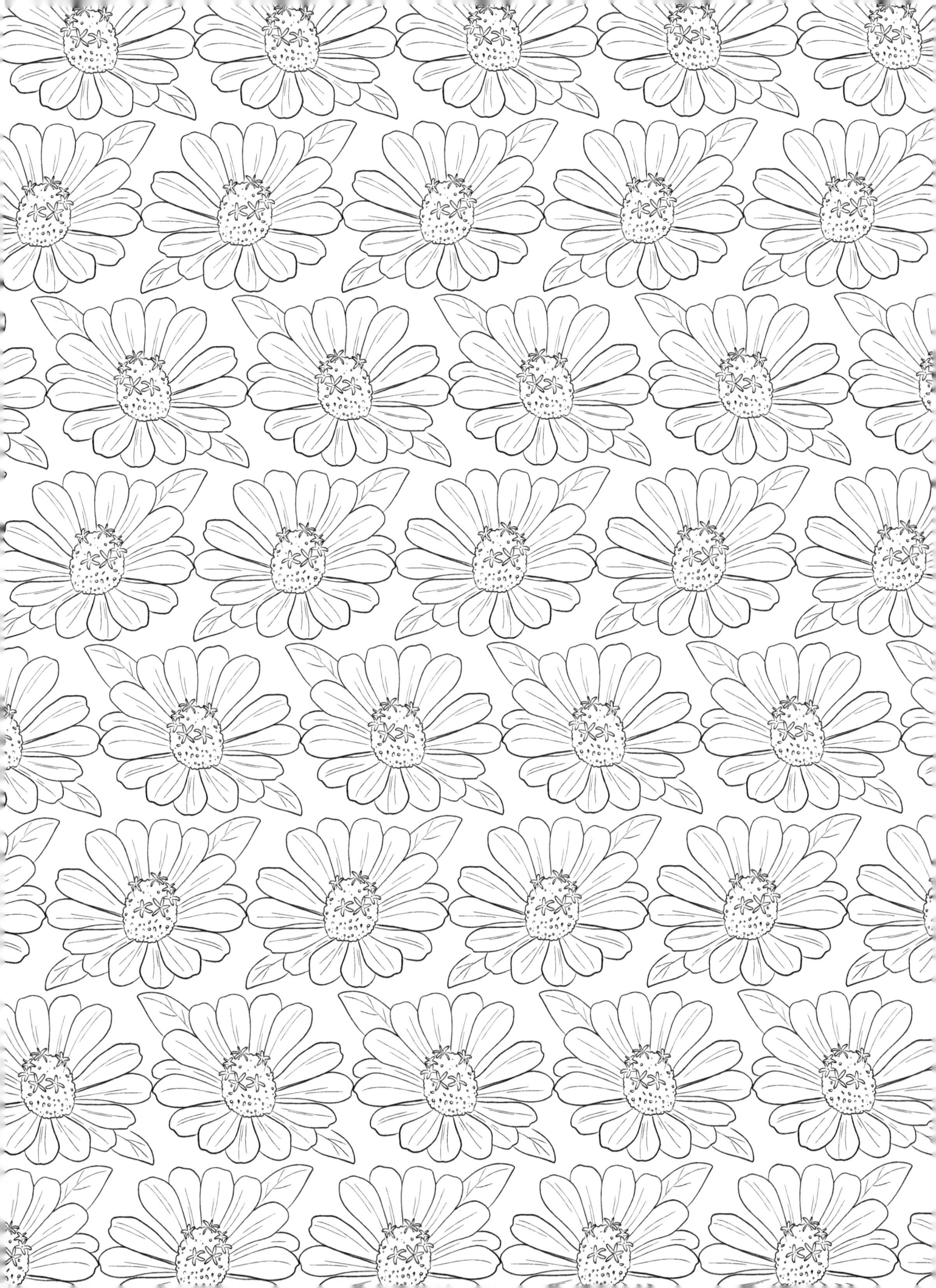

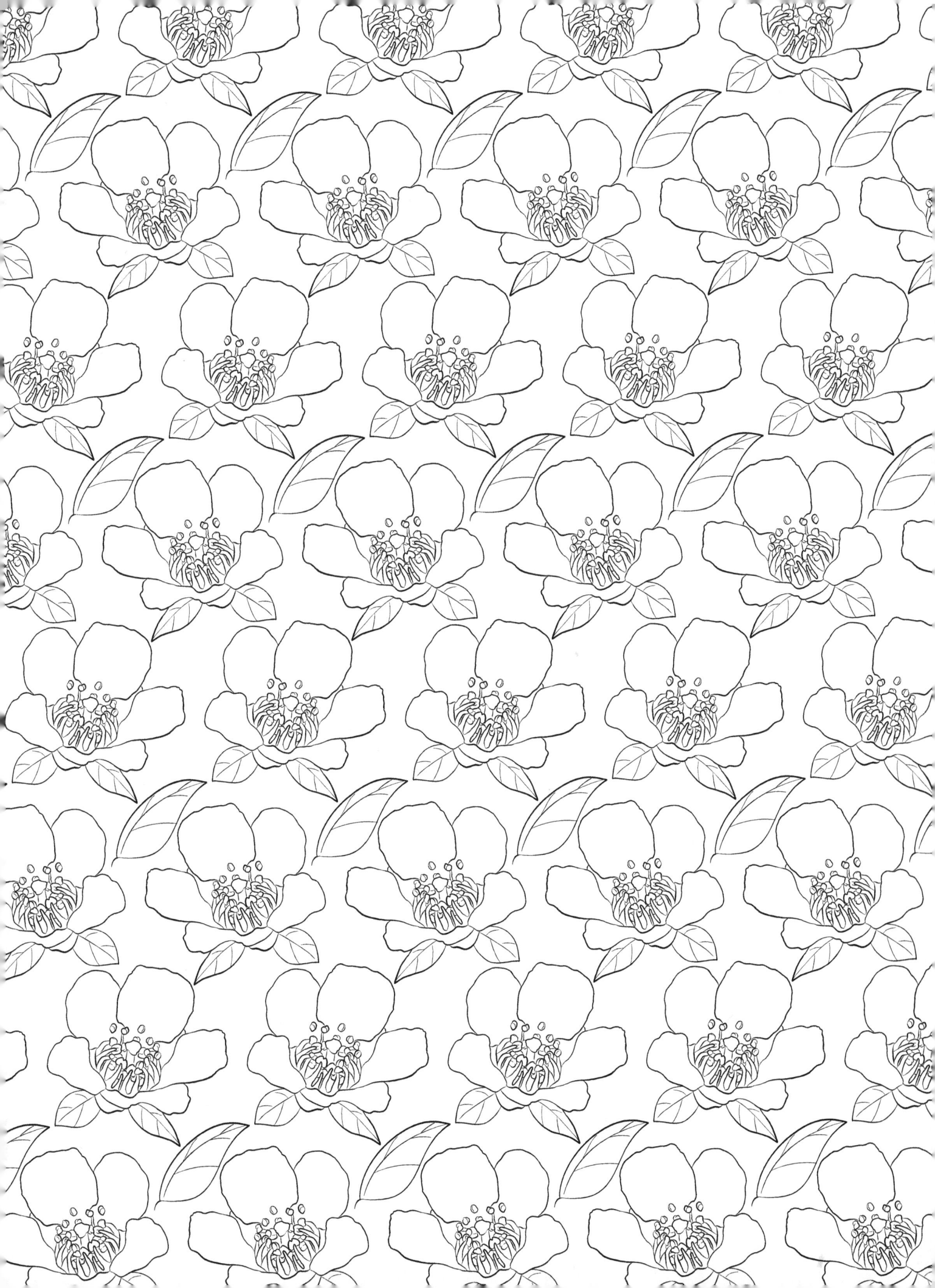

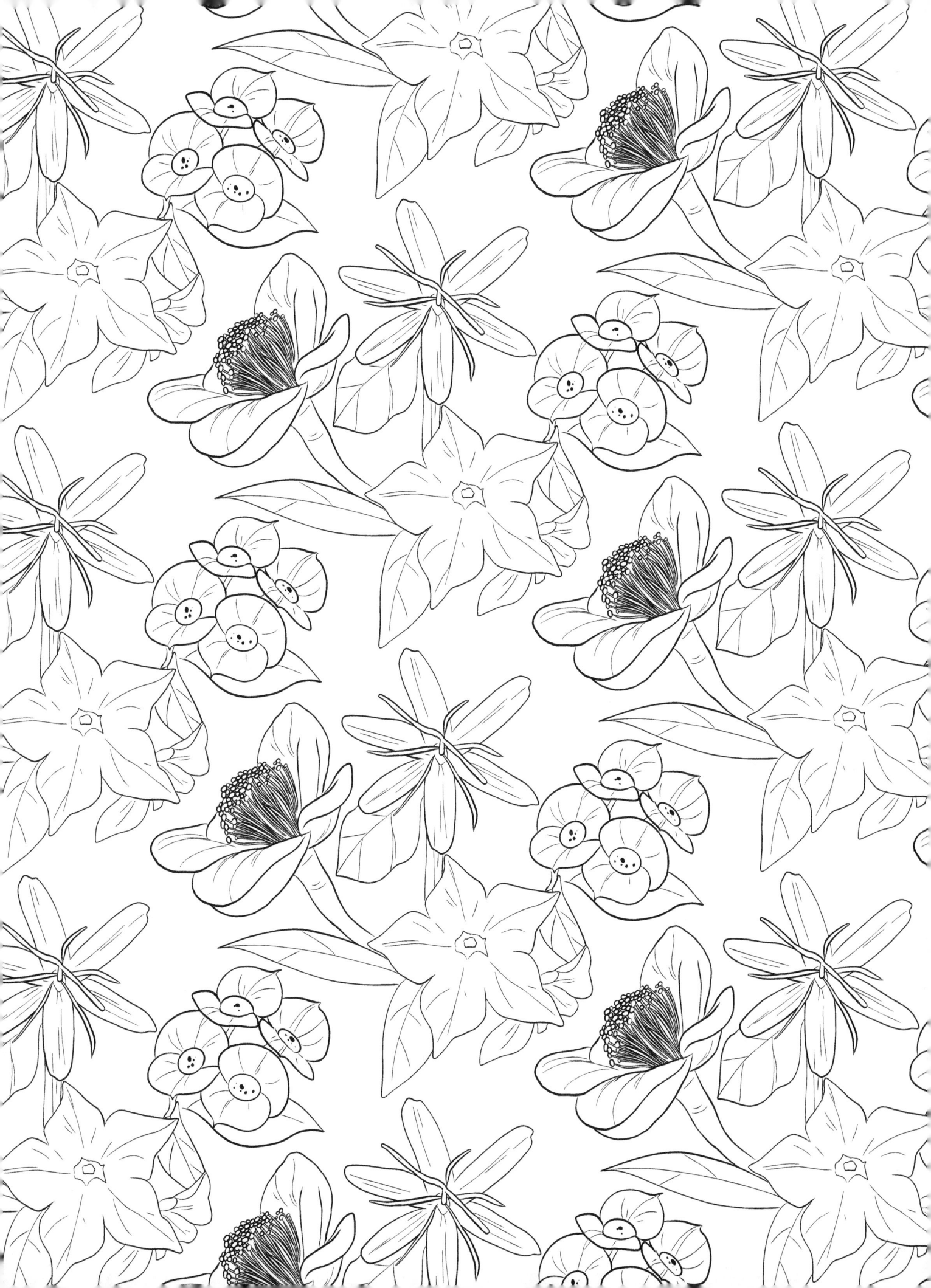

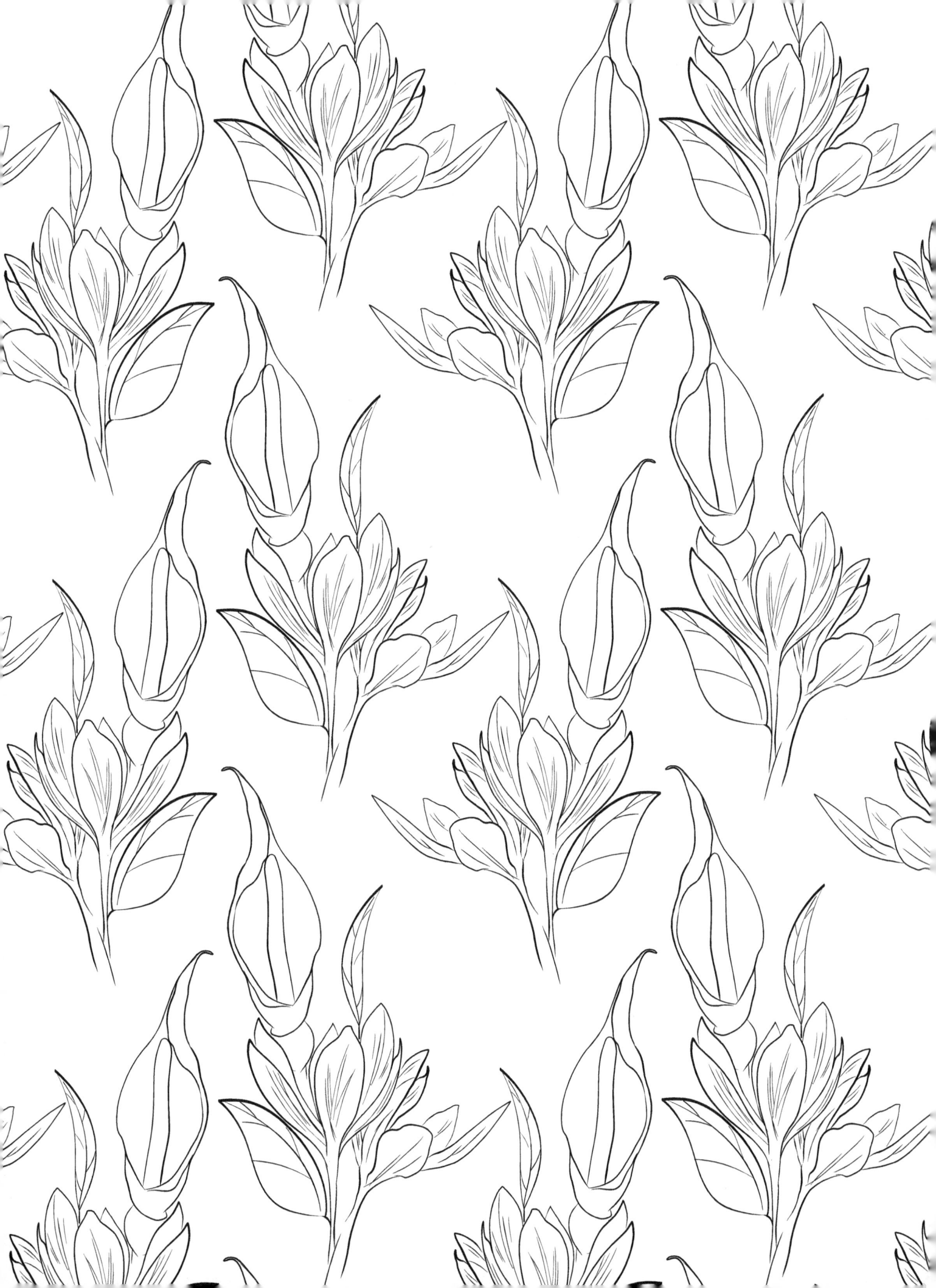

Scent Imagination

Look at the flower on the opposite page.

- Close your eyes
- Imagine the scent of this flower
- Imagine its color

The 60-Second Nature Scan

Look at the flower. Close your eyes and study its colors, textures, and shapes for 60 seconds. Now paint it as you imagined it.

Affirmation
Quote

Like a flower in sunlight,
I open gently to calm.

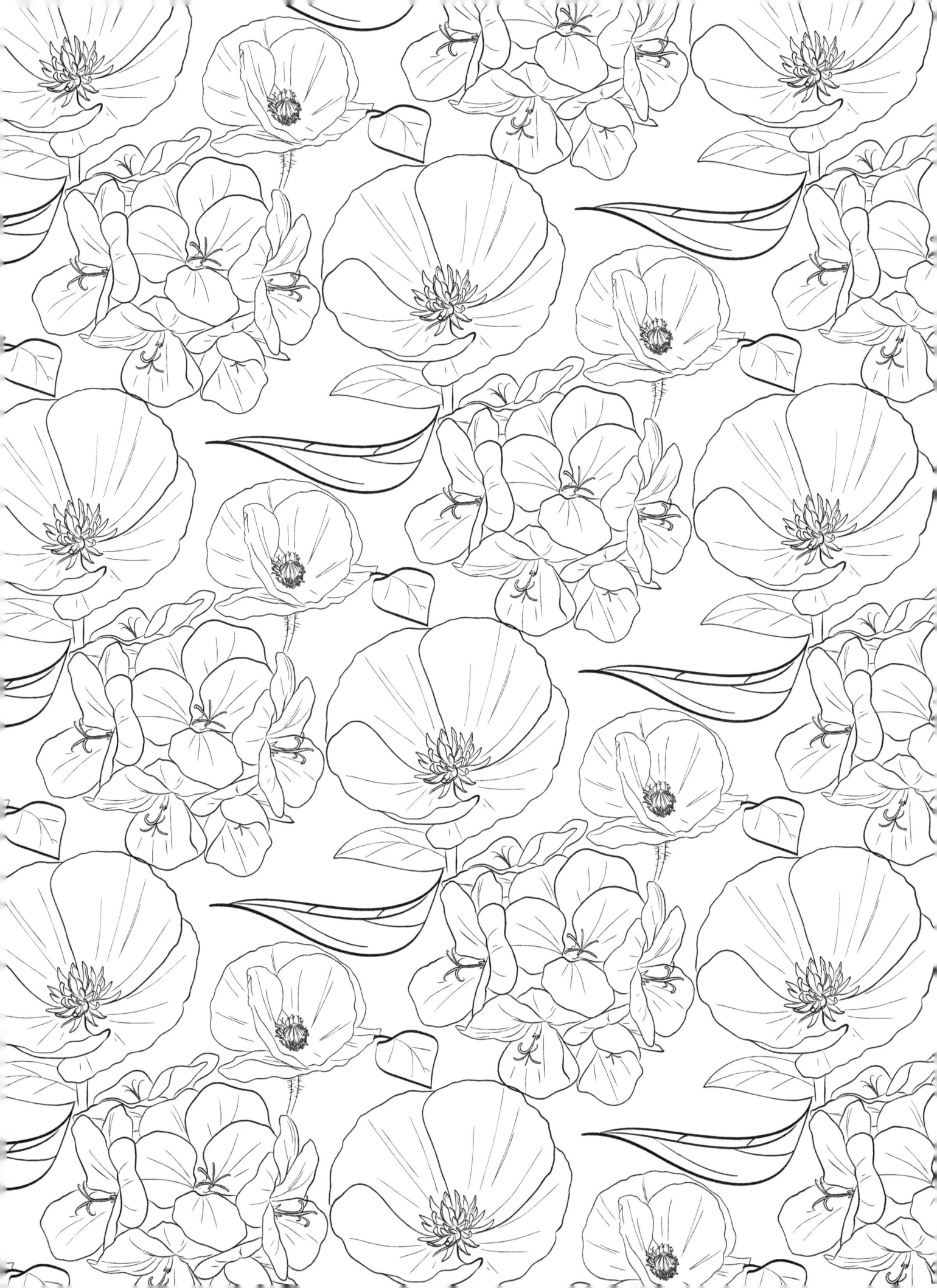

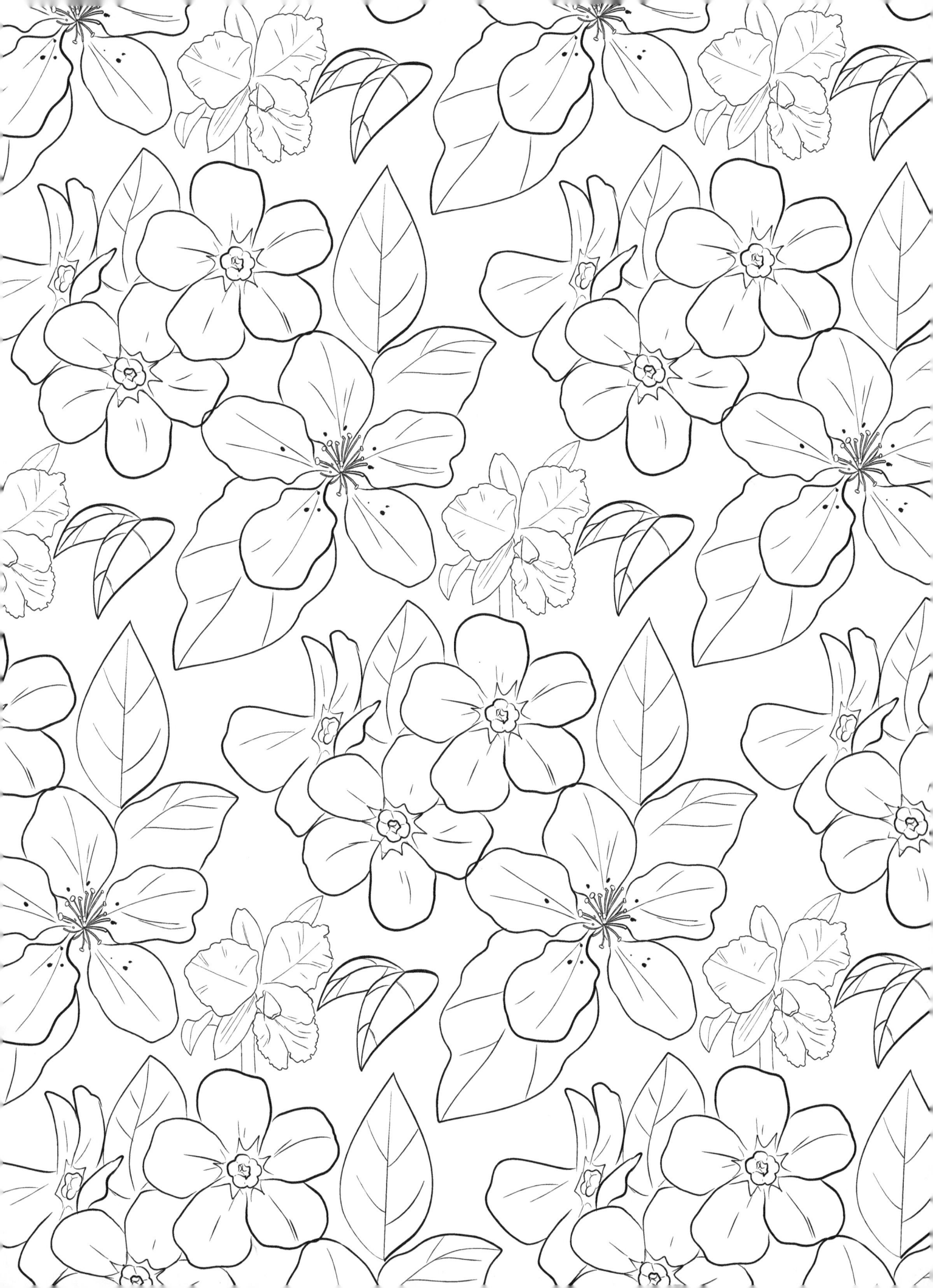

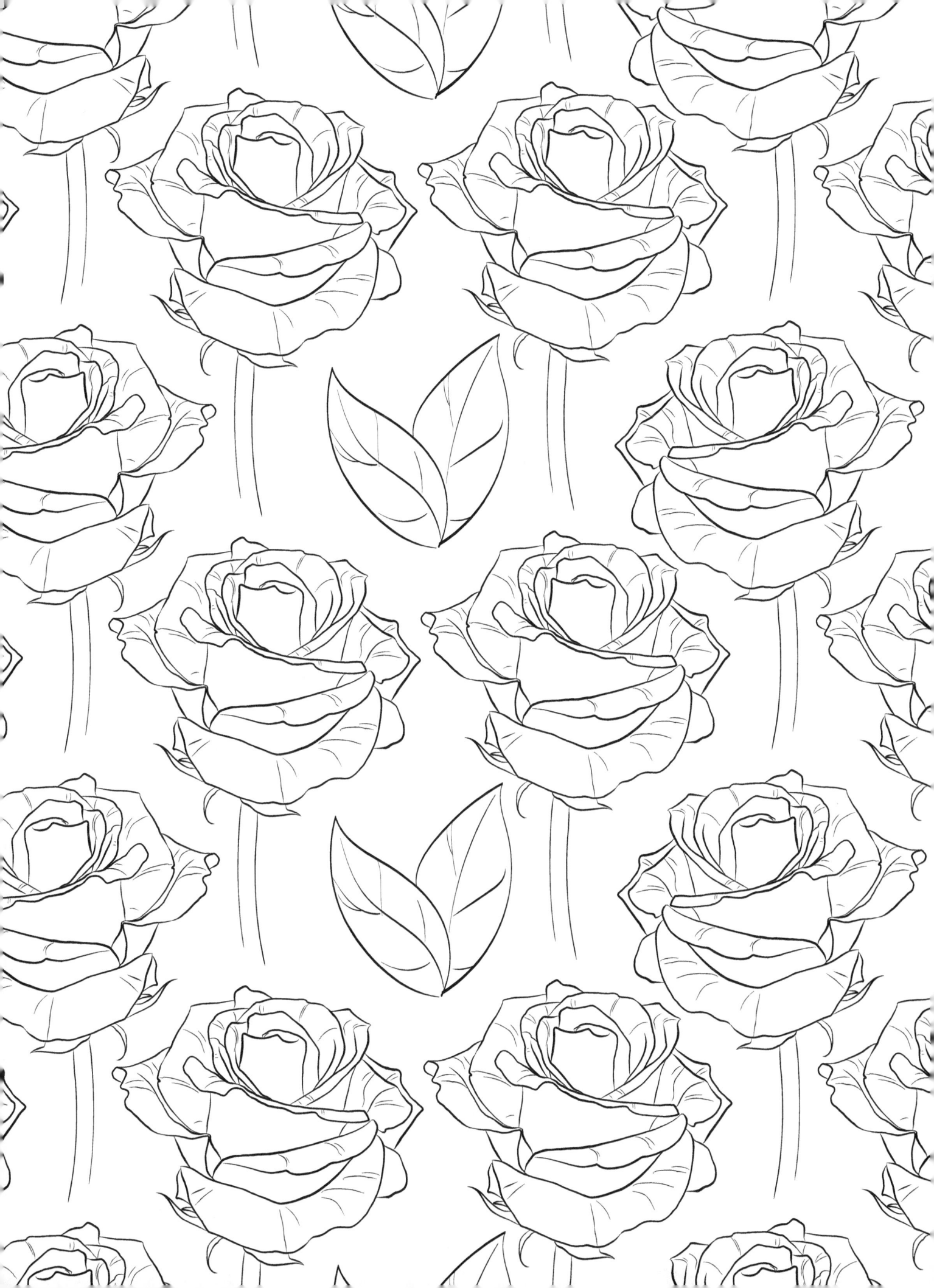

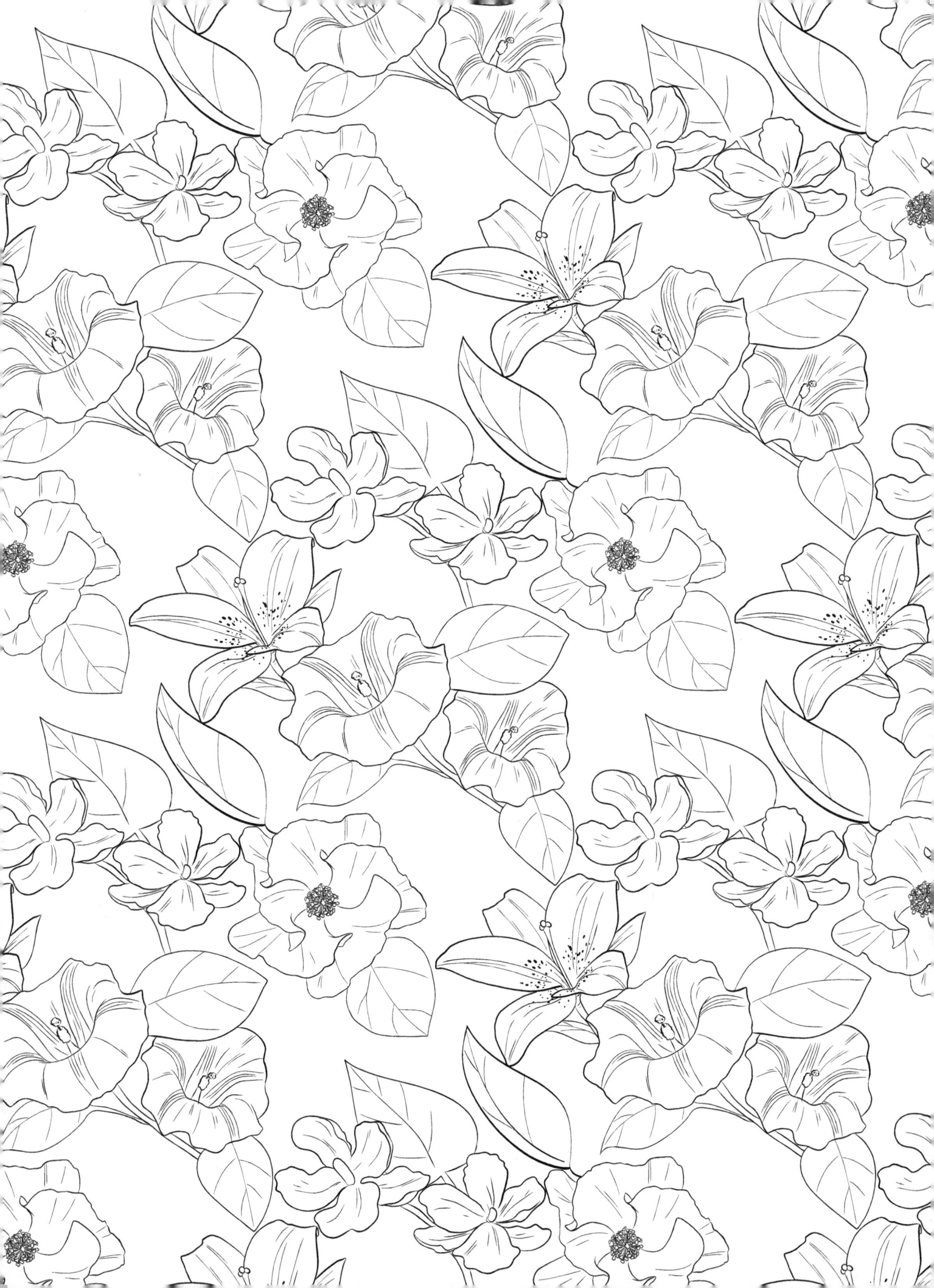

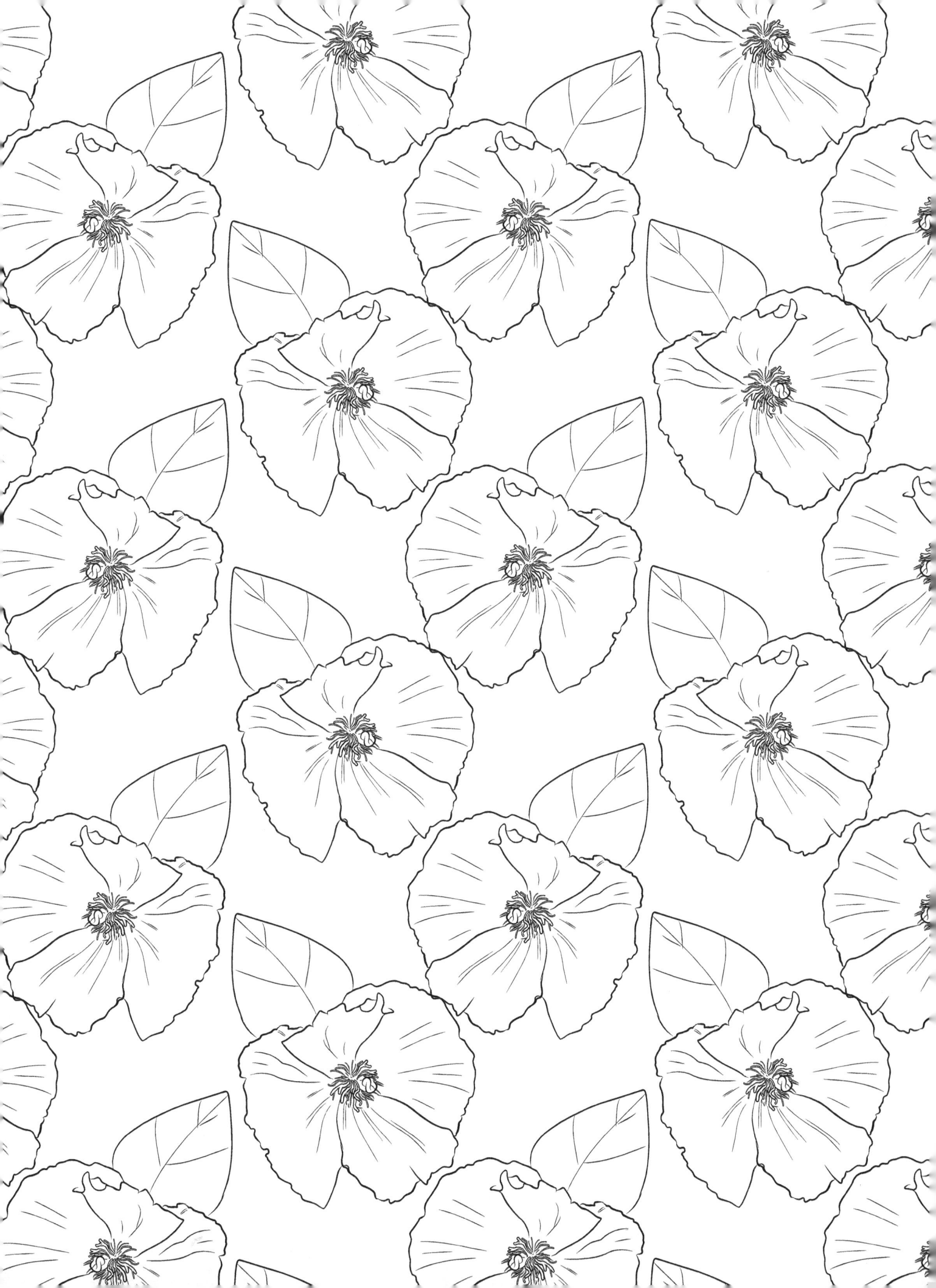

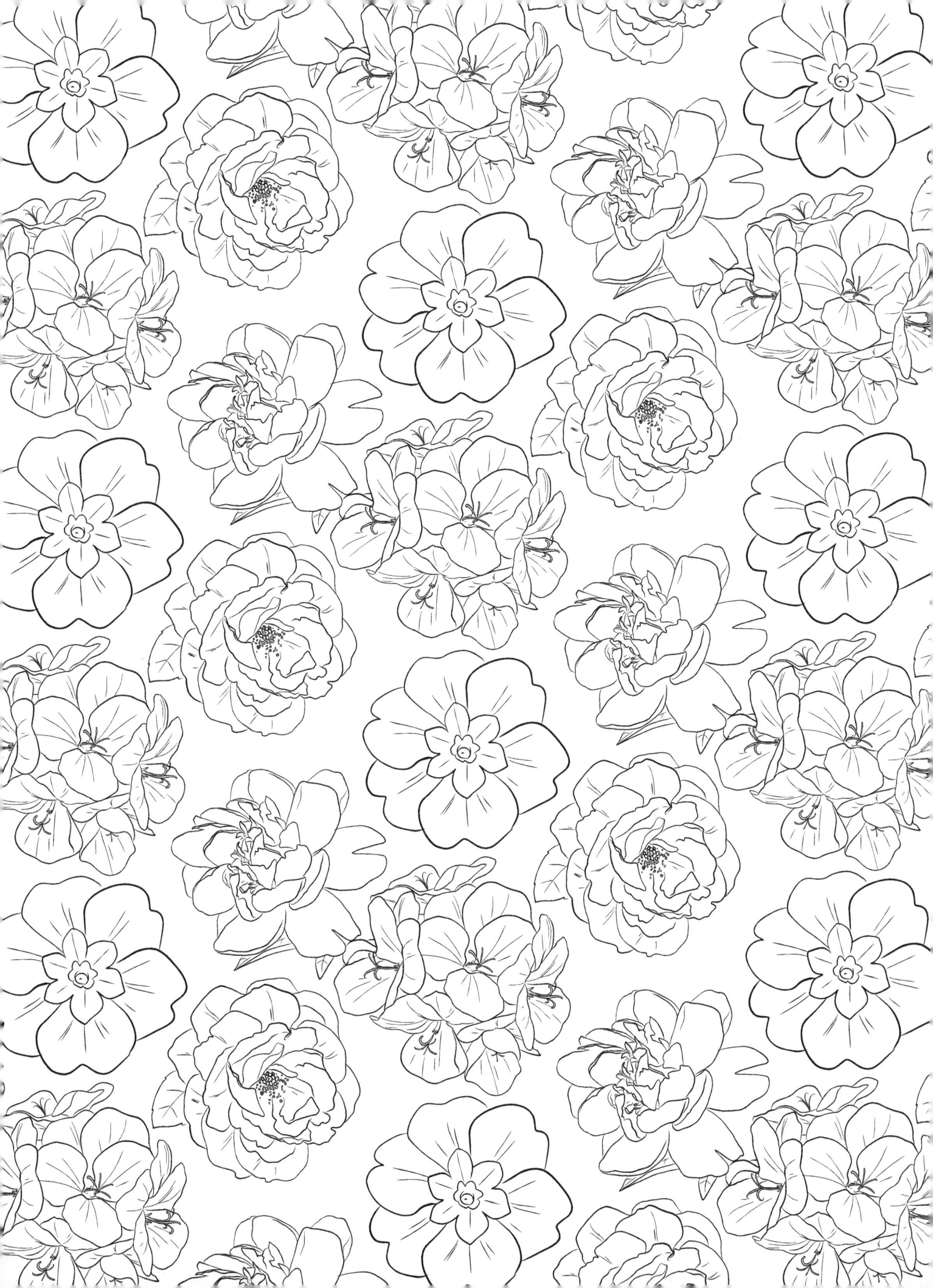

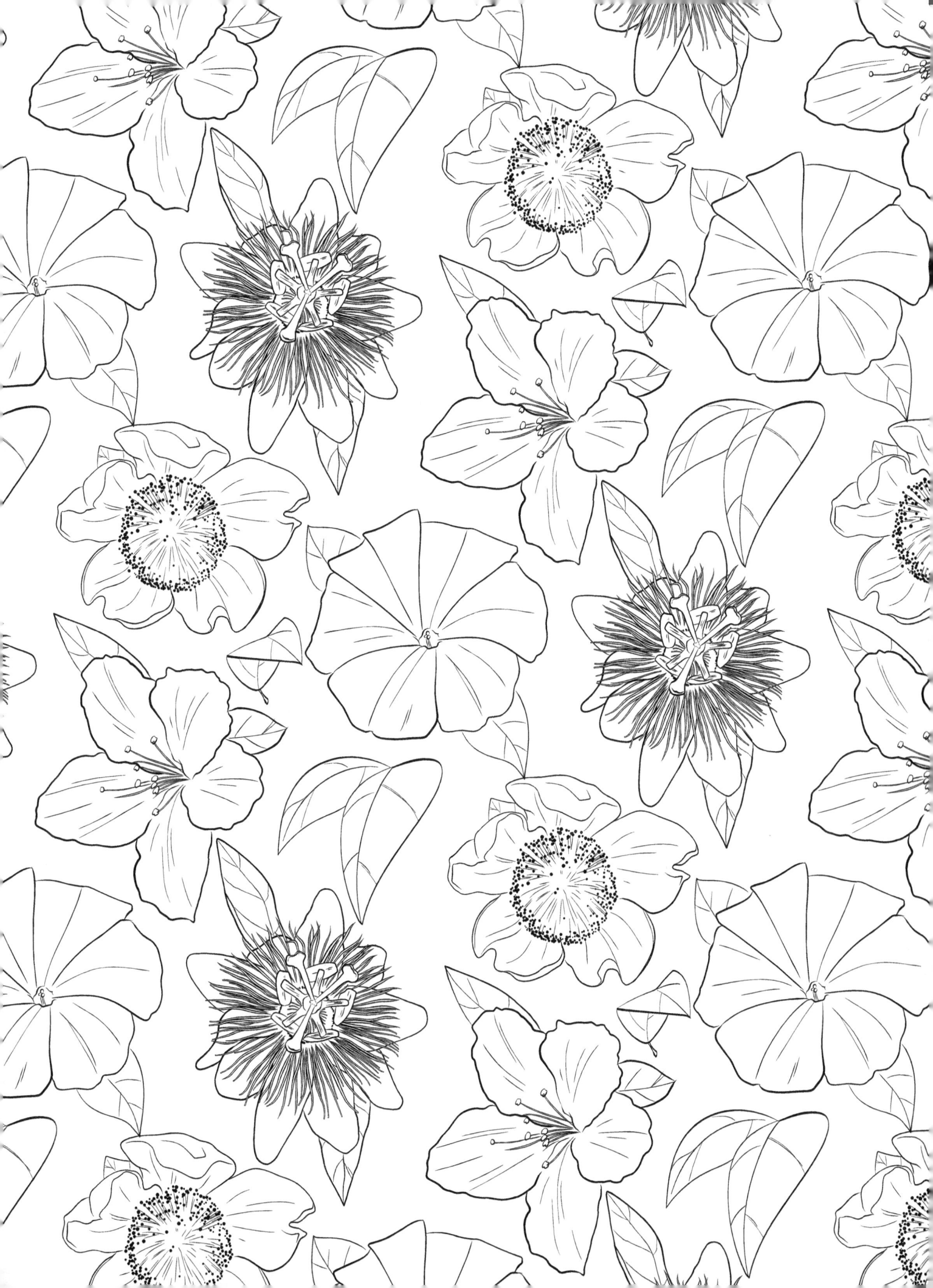

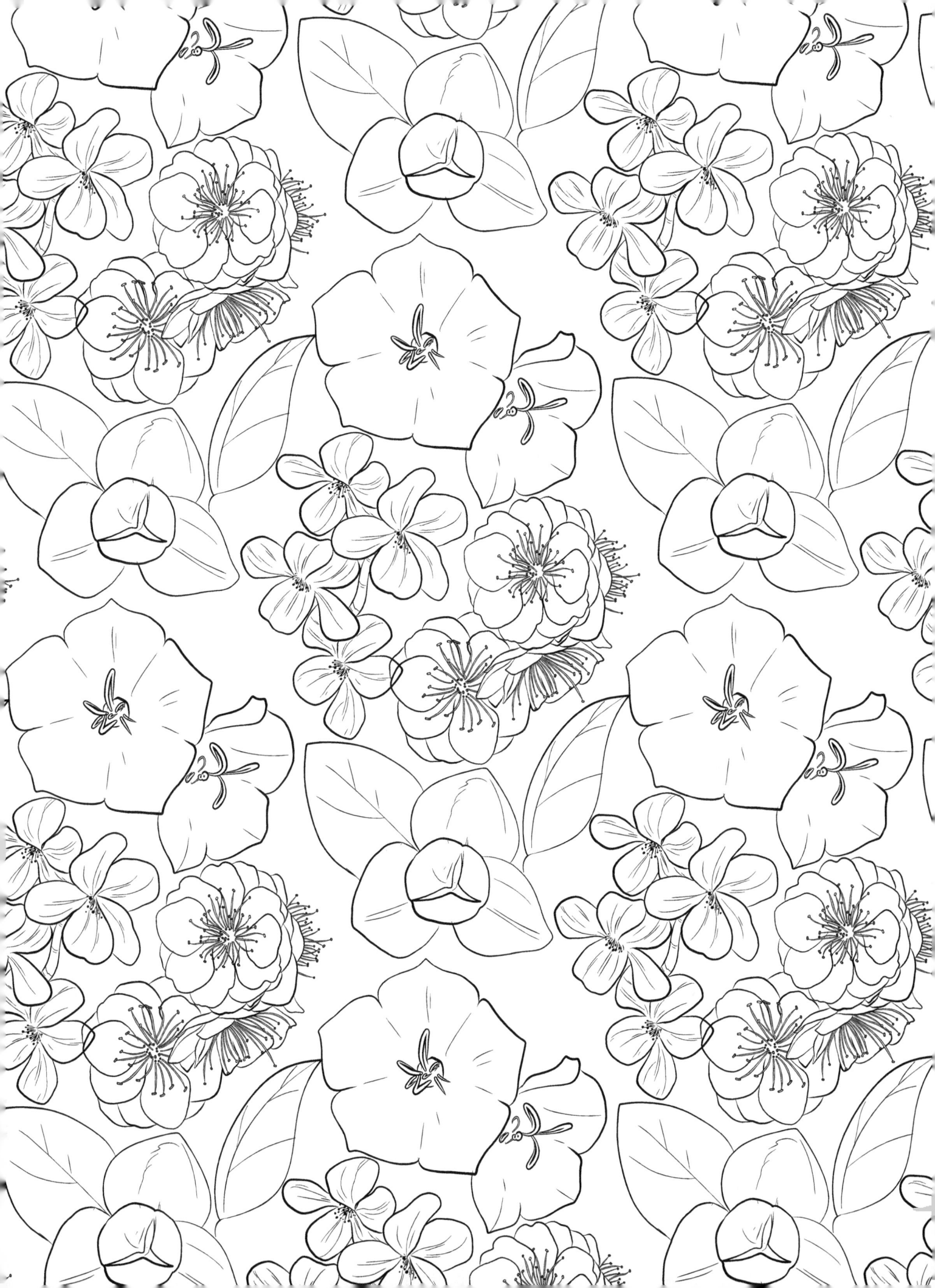

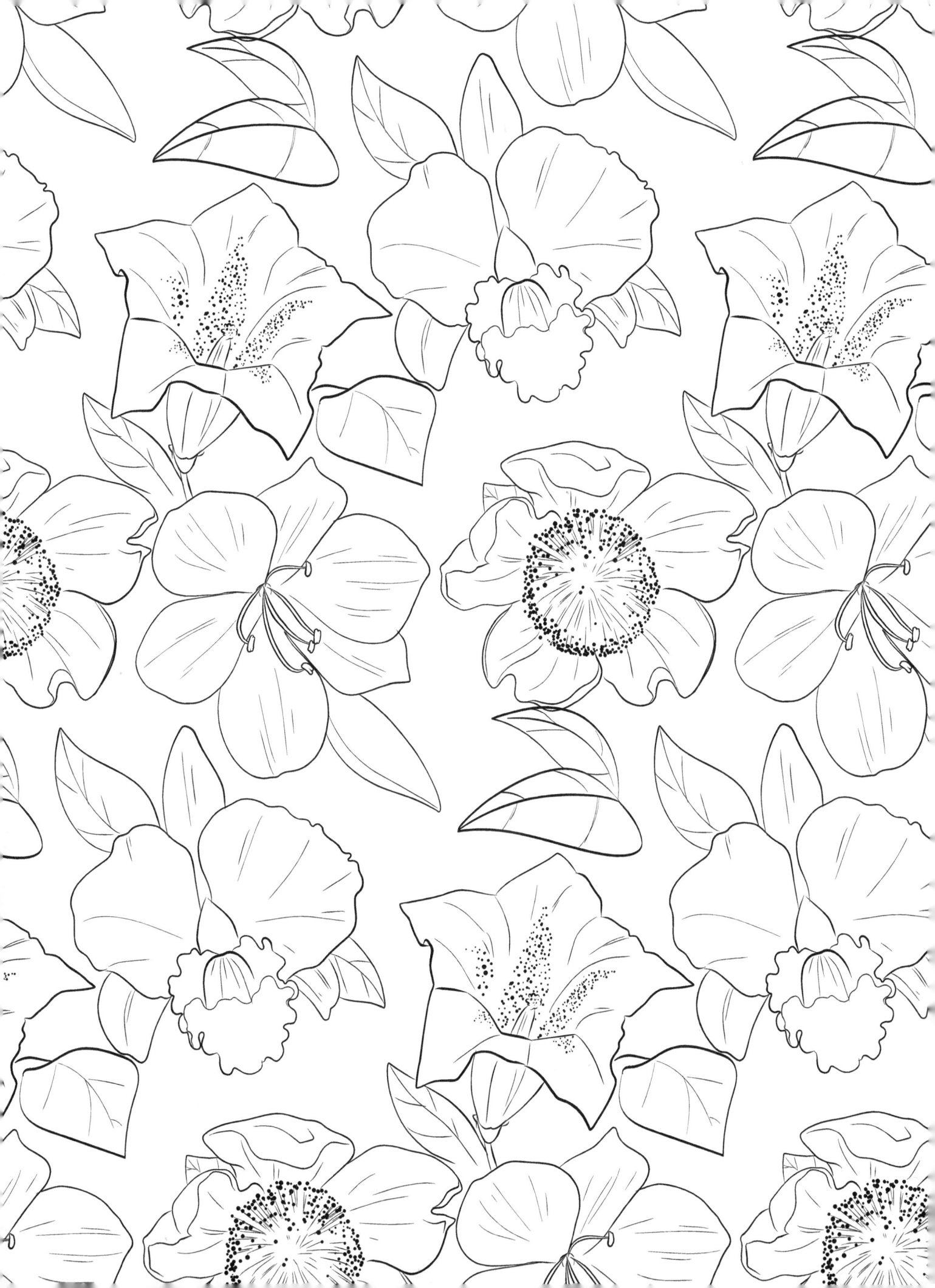

Scent Imagination

Look at the flower on the opposite page.

- Close your eyes
- Imagine the scent of this flower
- Imagine its color

The Breath Match Game

Breathe in for 4 counts, hold 4 counts, exhale for 4 counts, hold for 4 counts, and again, slowly and gently. Try to match the rhythm of your breath to a swaying flower blooming in the garden of your imagination.

Affirmation
Quote

I am allowed to pause.
I am allowed to breathe.

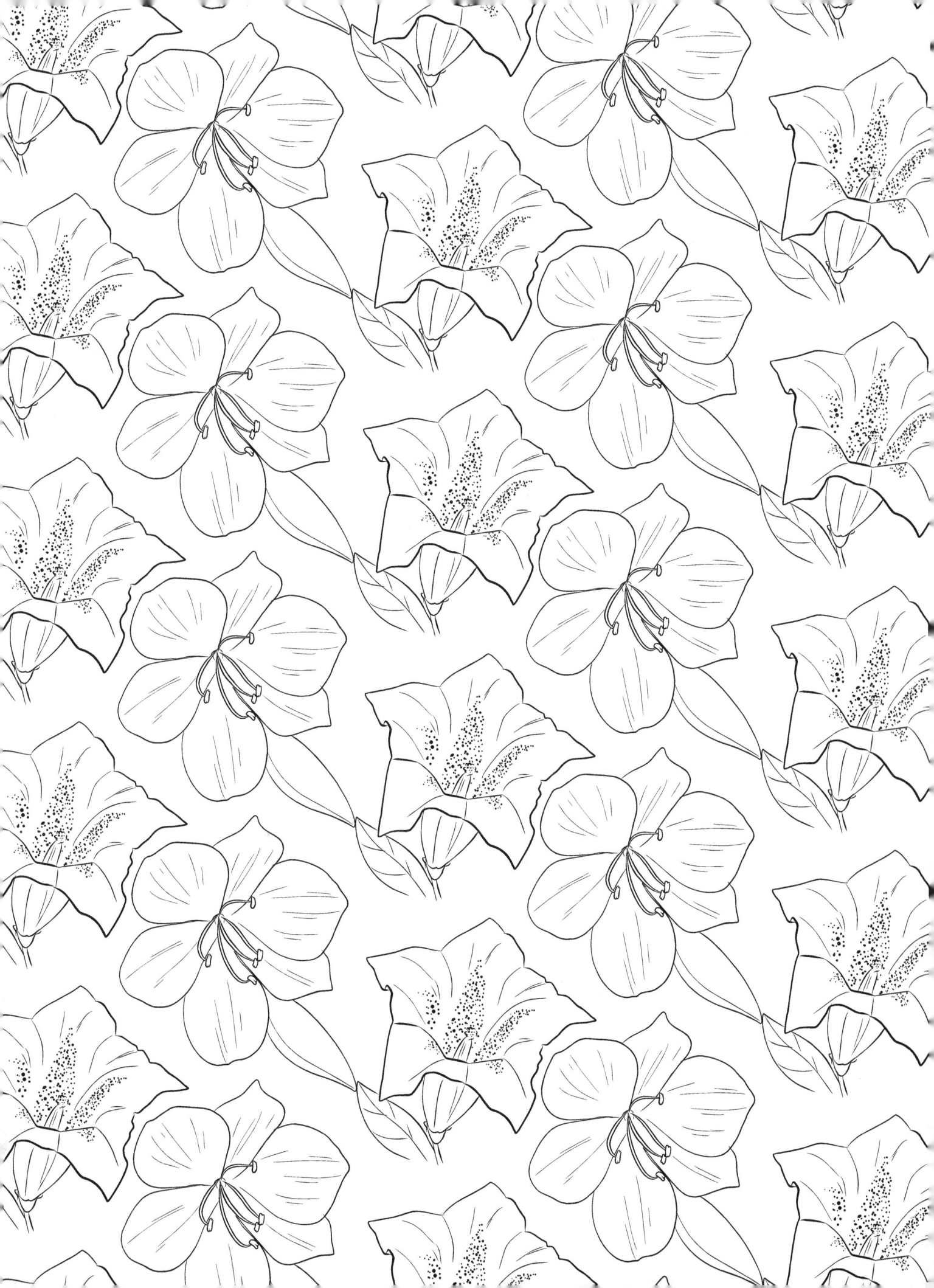

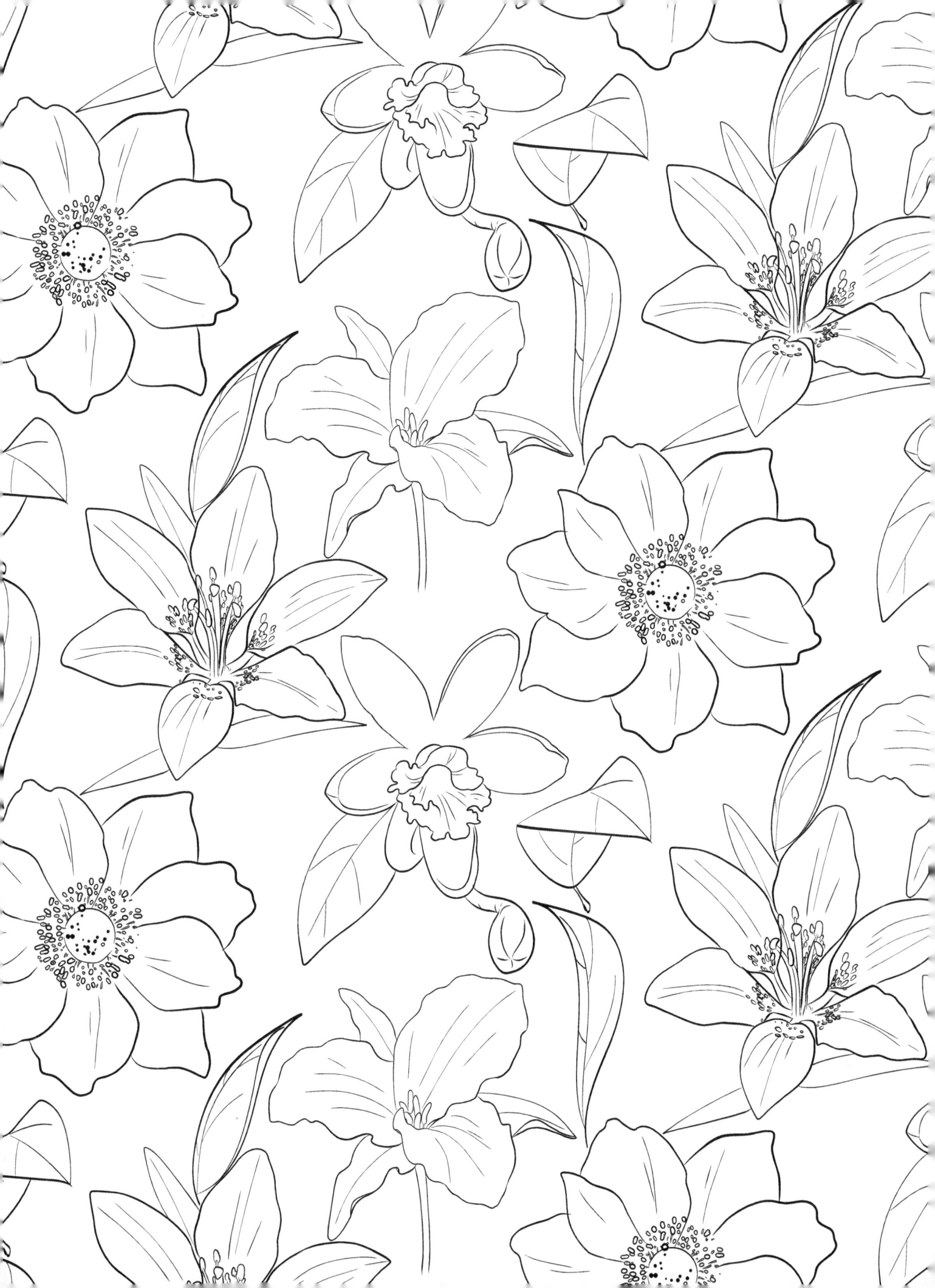

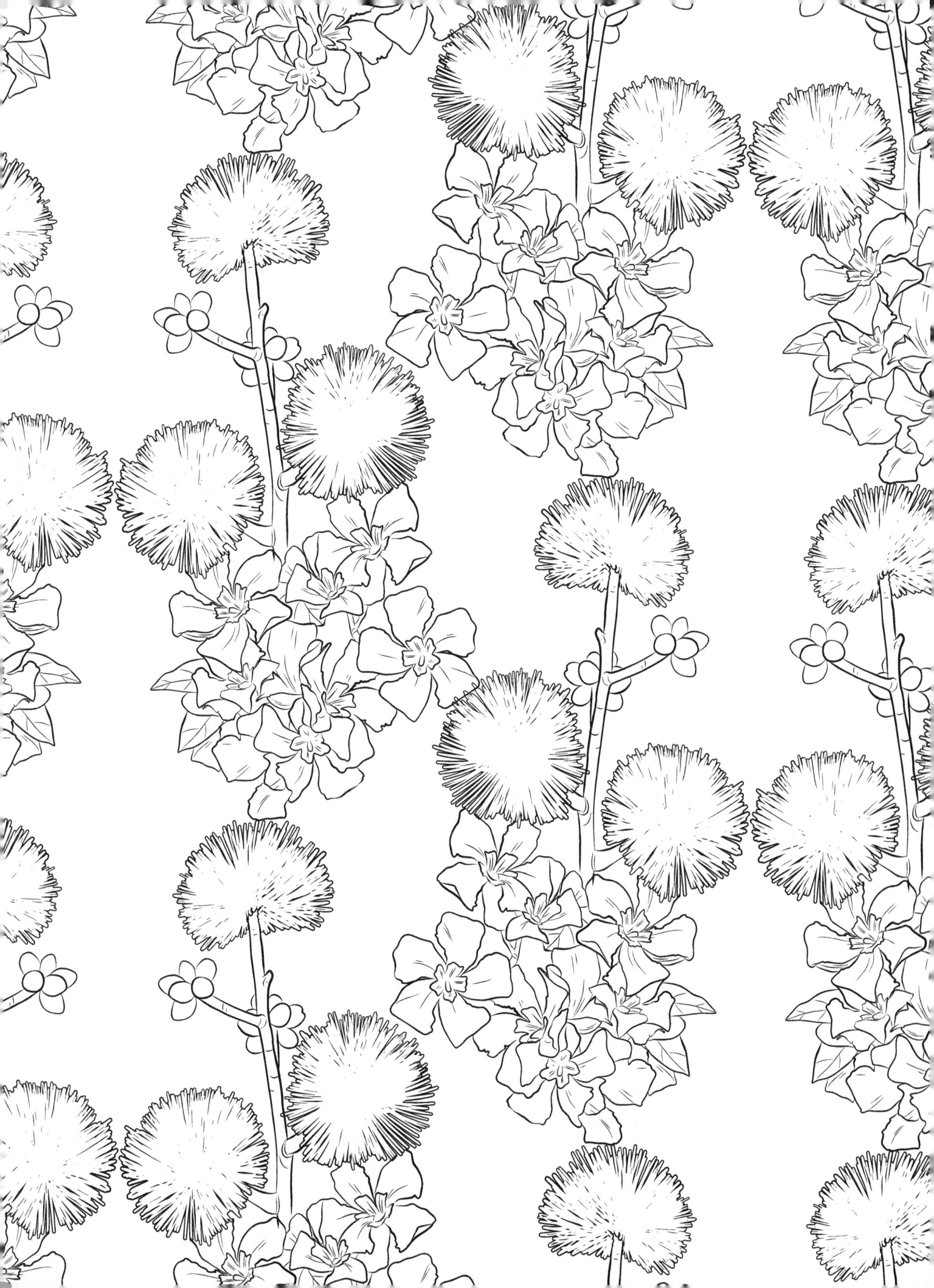

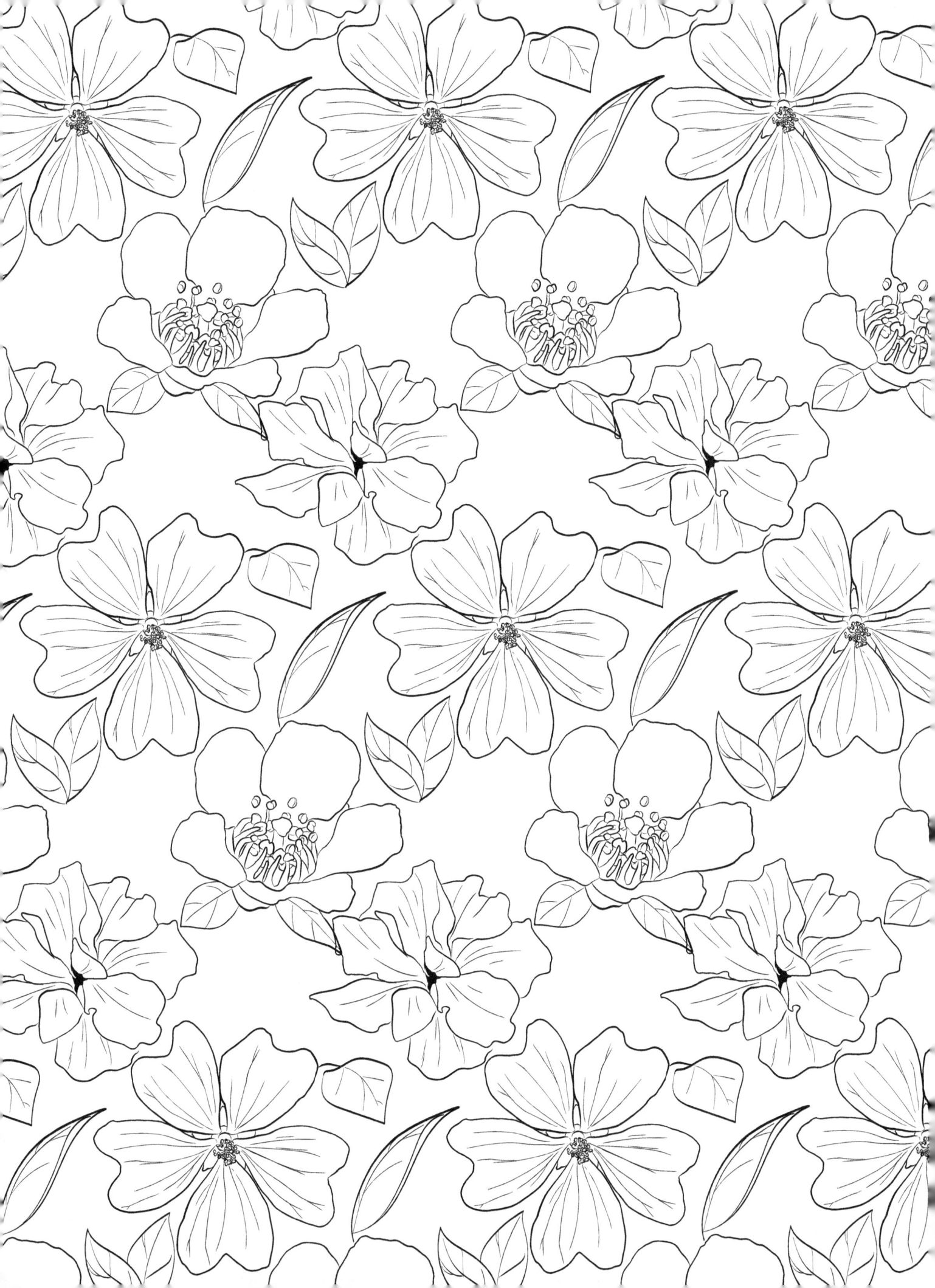

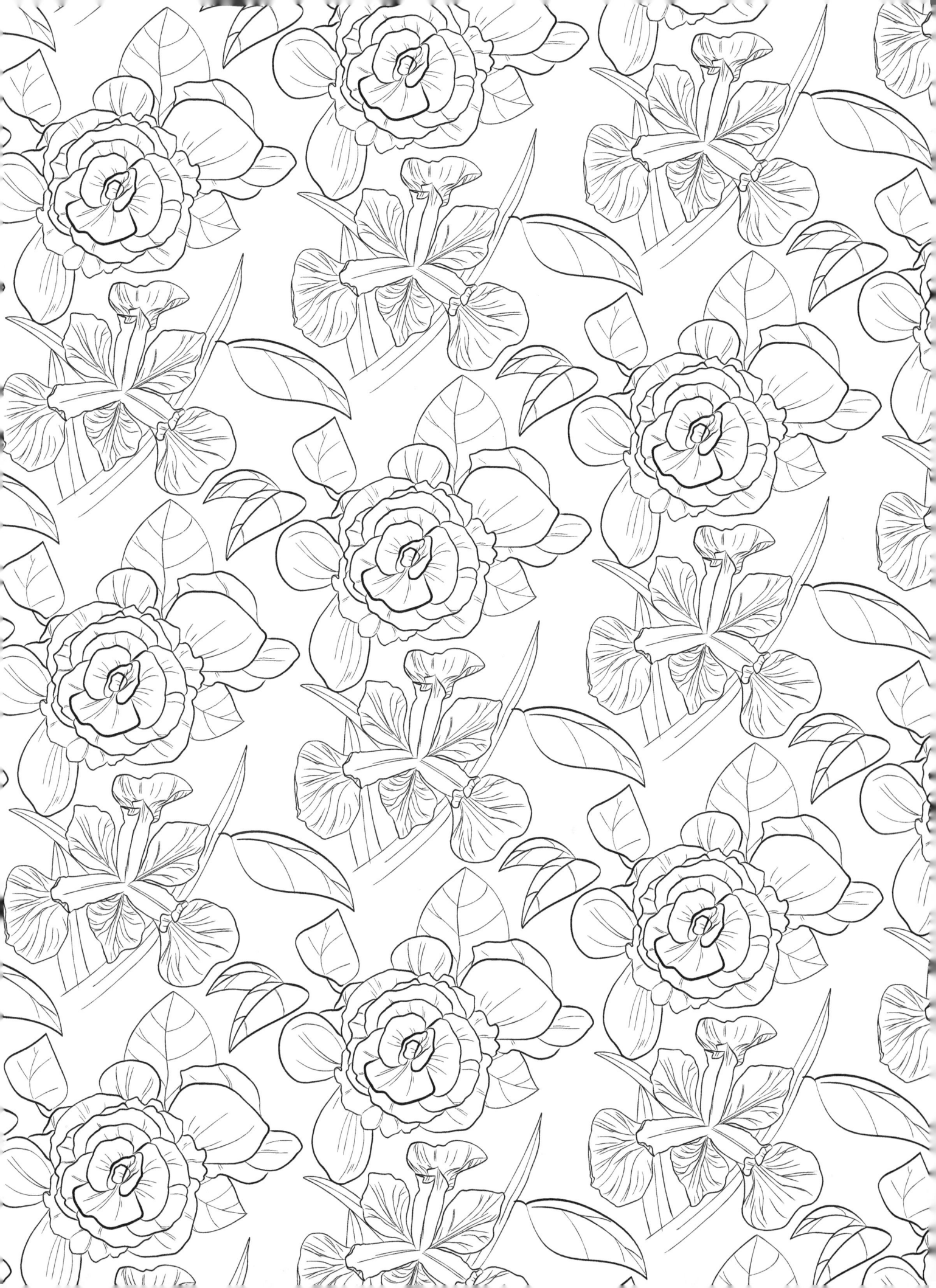

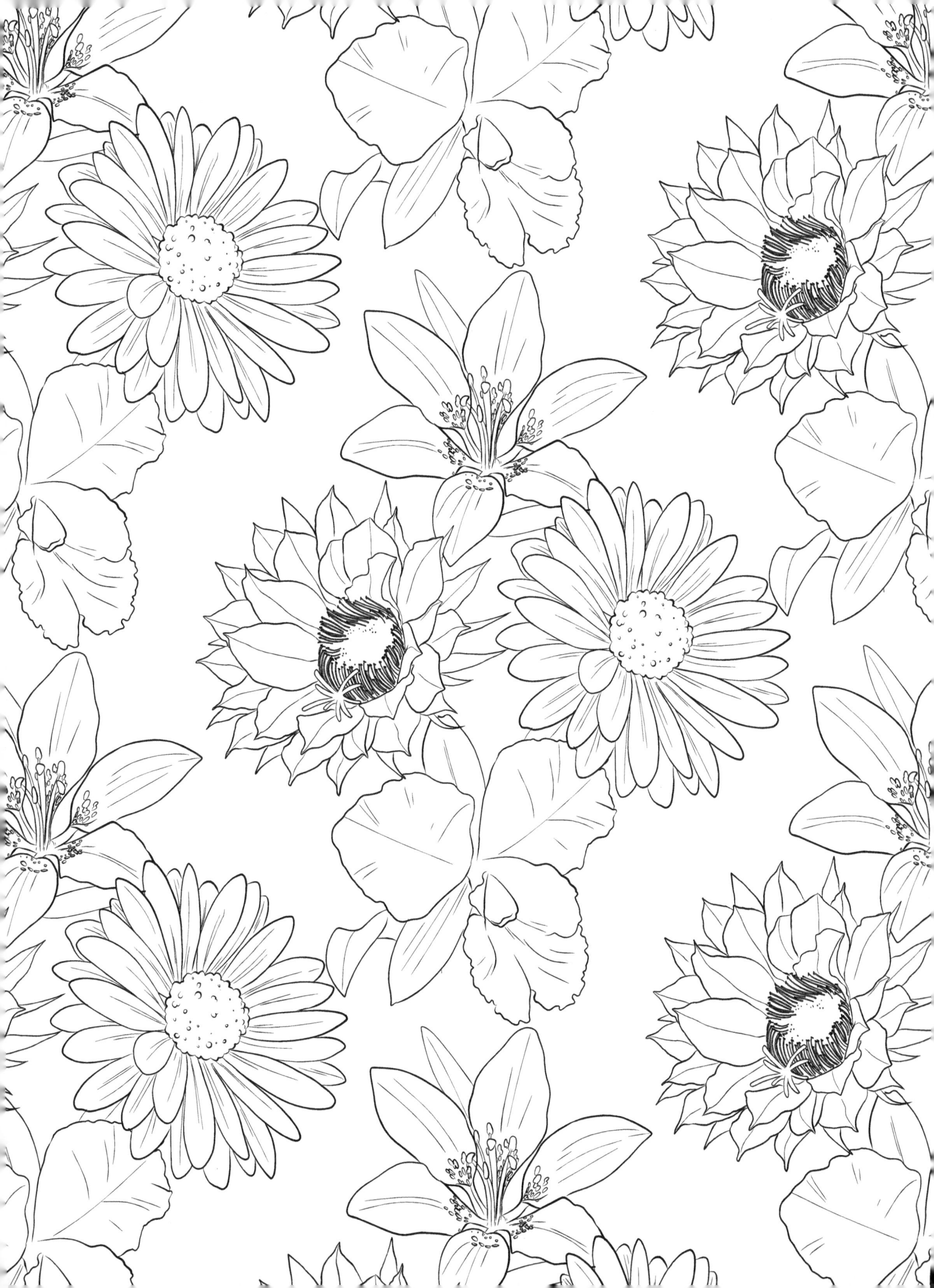

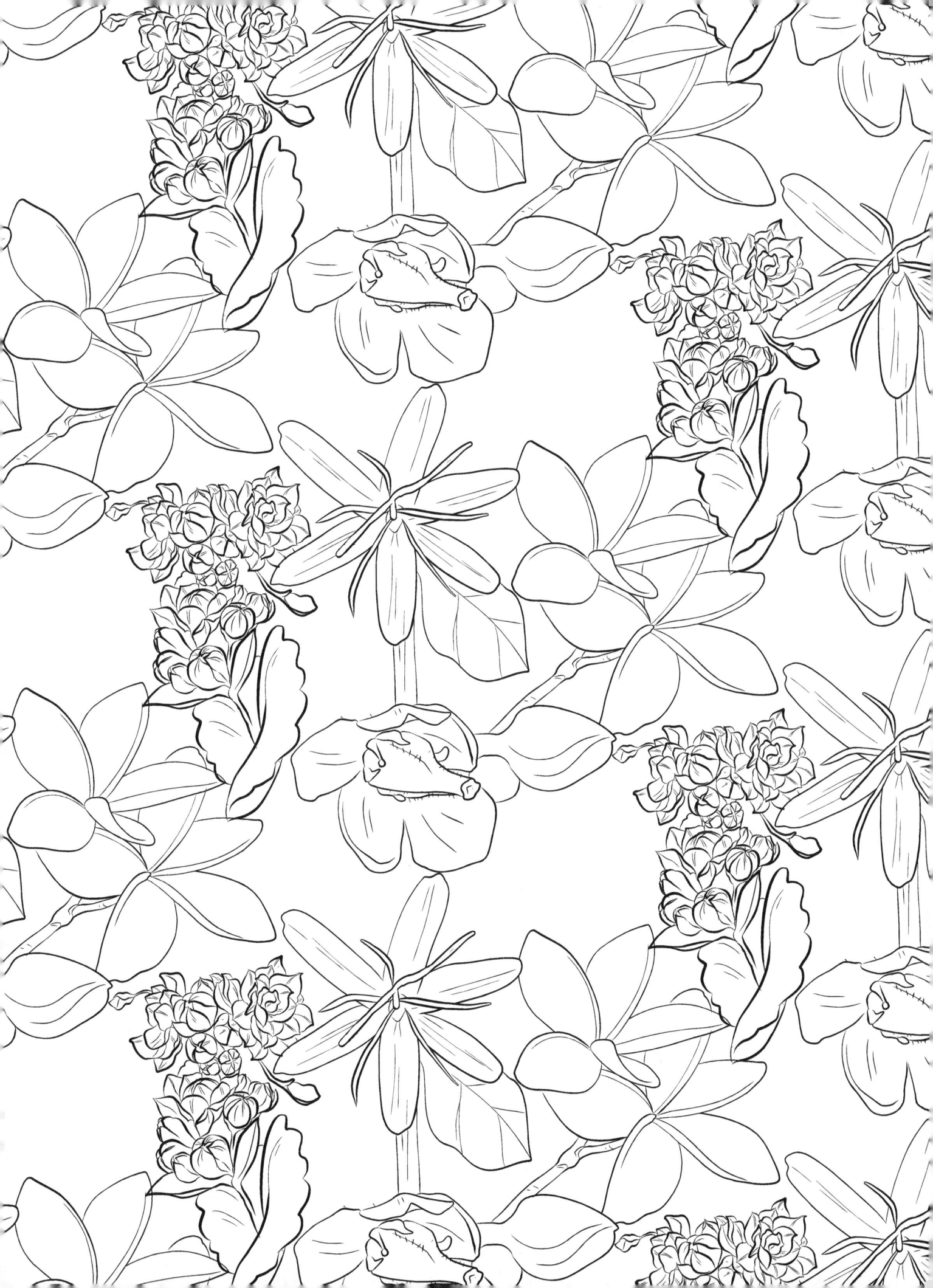

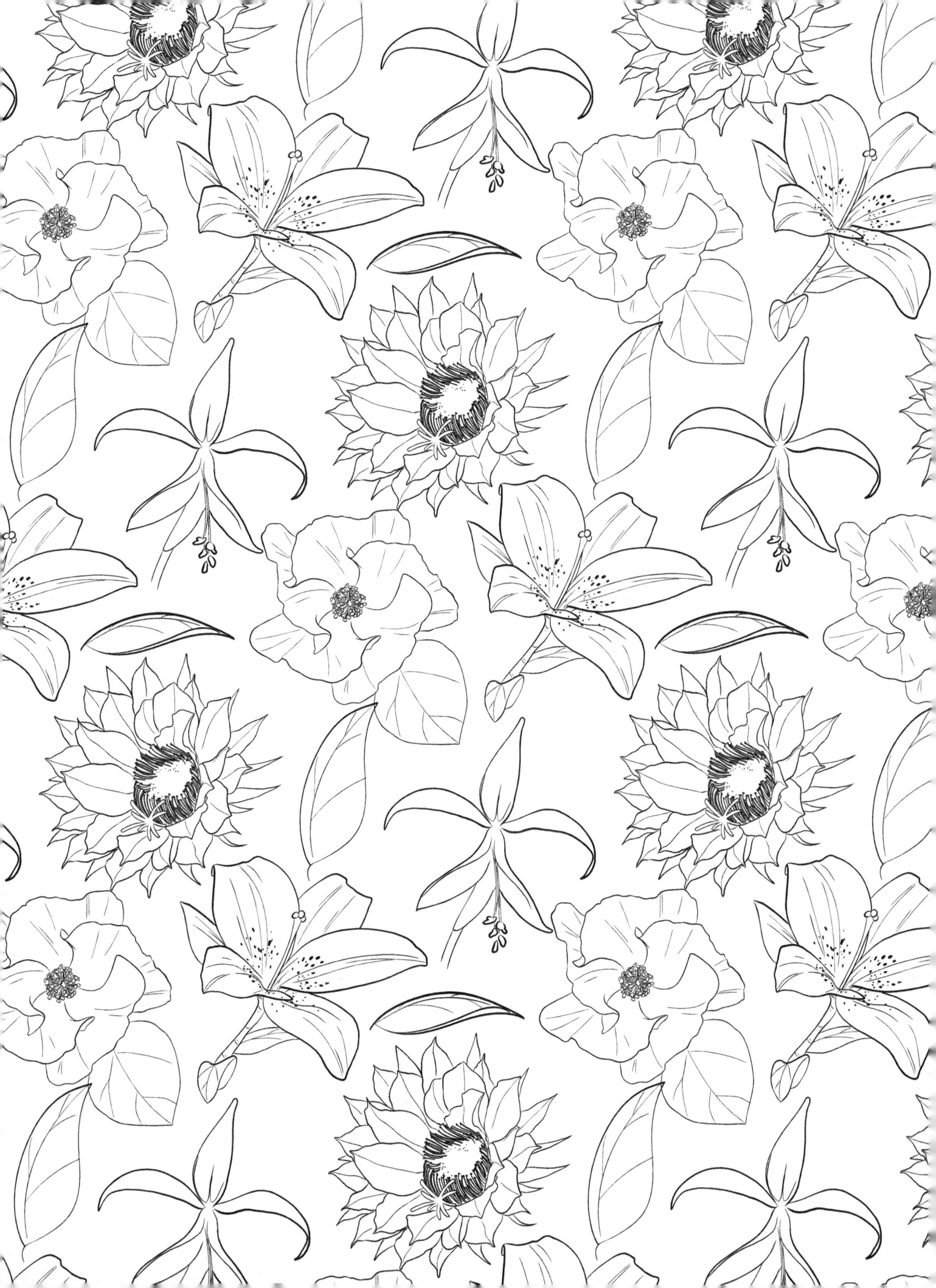

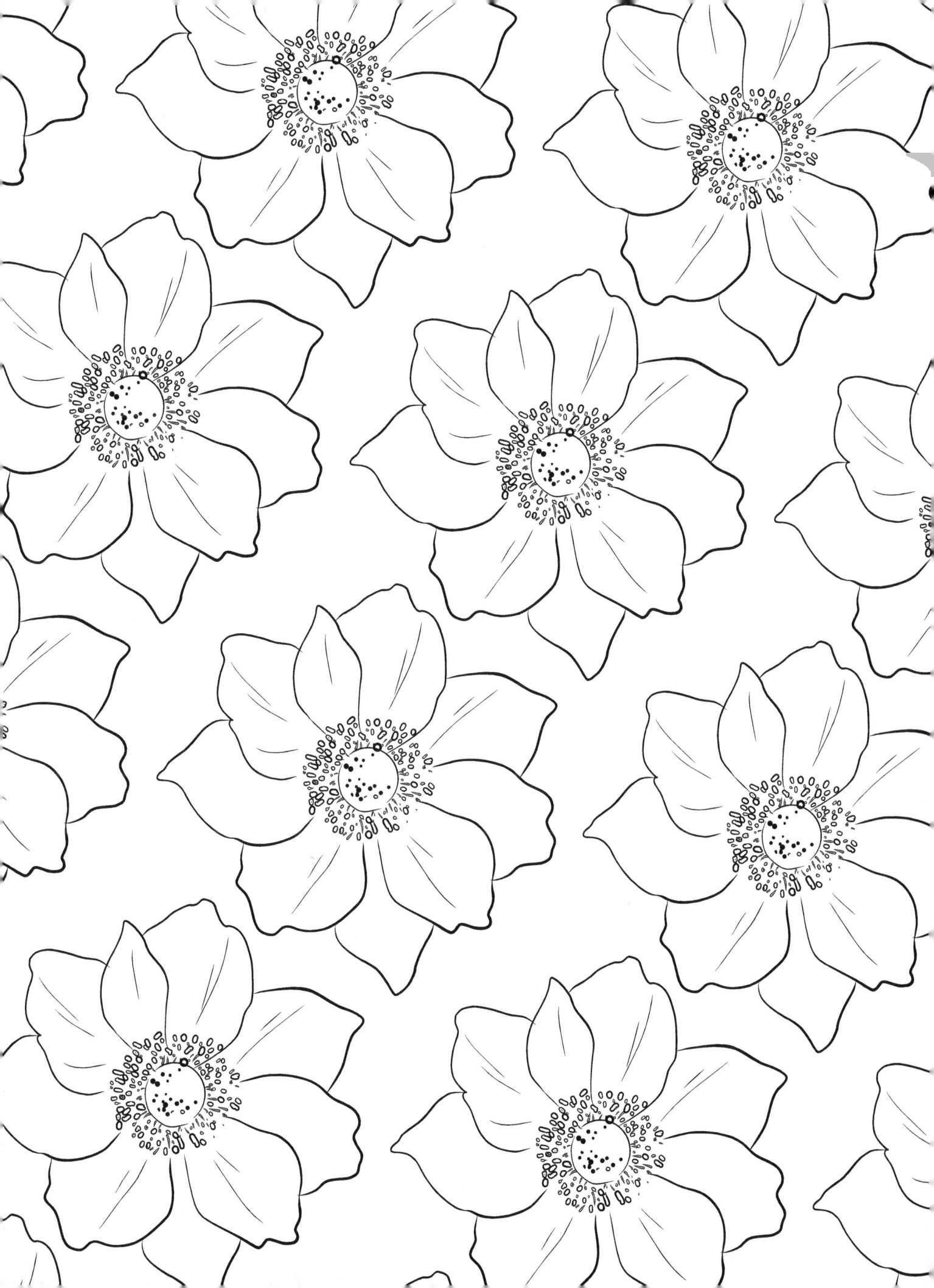

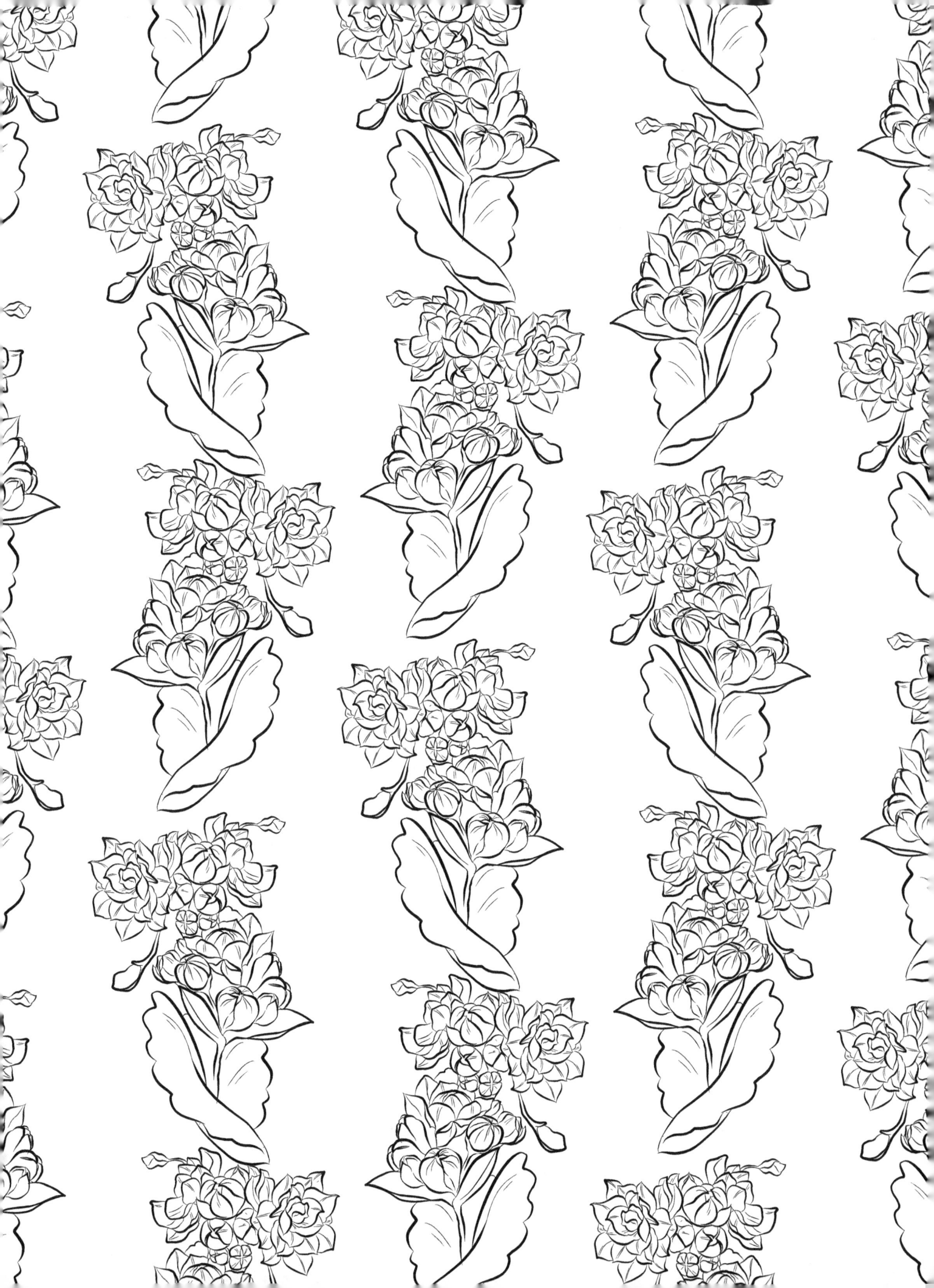

Peace

www.ingramcontent.com/pod-product-compliance
Lightning Source LLC
Chambersburg PA
CBHW081146020426
42333CB00021B/2686